Social Work Practice in Home Health Care

Social Work Practice in Home Health Care

Ruth Ann Goode, PhD

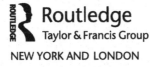

Routledge
Taylor & Francis Group

NEW YORK AND LONDON

First published 2000 by The Haworth Press, Inc.

Published 2009 by Routledge
605 Third Avenue, New York, NY 10017
4 Park Square, Milton Park, Abingdon, Oxon OX14 4RN

Routledge is an imprint of the Taylor & Francis Group, an informa business

Cover design by Jennifer M. Gaska.

Library of Congress Cataloging-in-Publication Data

Goode, Ruth Ann.
    Social work practice in home health care / Ruth Ann Goode.
        p.   cm.
    Includes bibliographical references and index.
    ISBN 0-7890-0483-6 (hardcover : alk. paper). — ISBN 0-7890-0484-4 (pbk. : alk. paper)
    1. Medical social work—United States. 2. Home care services—United States. I. Title.
HV687.5.U5G66 1999
362.1'0425—dc21   99-37682
                                                                                    CIP

Publisher's Note
The publisher has gone to great lengths to ensure the quality of this reprint but points out that some imperfections in the original may be apparent.

ISBN 13: 978-0-7890-0484-0 (pbk)

CONTENTS

ABOUT THE AUTHOR

Ruth Ann Goode, PhD, LISW, ACSW, is a licensed independent social worker for Aware Resources, Inc. in Cuyahoge Falls, Ohio. She also provides home health care consultation, training, and education. Dr. Goode has held adjunct teaching positions in psychology at Notre Dame College in Cleveland and Park College in Newark, Ohio. She has conducted numerous workshops and seminars and has authored professional papers on gerontological and medical social work issues. Dr. Goode is listed in *Who's Who Among American Women* and *Who's Who Among Human Service Professionals.* She is also a member of the National Association of Social Workers and the Academy of Certified Social Workers.

Foreword

Two realities are slowly being accepted in the United States: one is demographic and the other is procedural. The first is that the aging population is a large and increasing segment. The second is that care delivery is really evolving into a system.

This book appears at an opportune juncture. Long-established processes are being examined and amended. Long-term care agencies are exploring how social work services can both maximize care delivery and be a financial benefit.

This work represents the transformation of an academic study into an applied practitioner guide. All social and health care professionals—including physicians, HMO executives, and long-term care administrators—need to read and study this book. It will become a seminal reference work to be consulted for many years.

Marcia B. Steinhauer, PhD
Associate Professor
and Coordinator of Human Services
Administration Program
Rider University
Lawrenceville, New Jersey

Preface

It has been almost two decades since I began practicing social work. This very important role has given me the opportunity to listen to and work with clients of all ages, backgrounds, and problems. Over the past decade, I have been practicing social work in the home health care field. I have seen clients in their natural environments and their support systems. This privileged position has allowed me to practice grassroots social work on inner-city streets, in suburbia, and in rural America. I have seen abuse, neglect, poverty, malnutrition, uninhabitable housing, dysfunctional families, sensory deprivation, isolation, caregiver stress, alcohol and drug abuse, and clients in need of community resources to better cope with their life situations. Over the course of my doctoral research, I became interested in the area of social work practice in home health agencies, and it became the focus of my research. Through the interests of Walden University faculty and my adviser, Dr. Marcia Steinhauer, and support from my friend Carol Eldridge, this book has become a reality. I would also like to thank Theresa Lydonne Wilson for the preparation of the entire manuscript.

At this writing, home health care is at a crucial crossroads with the emergence of managed care, prospective pay, fraud, abuse, and cost reductions. It is my sincere hope that during this financial crisis facing the industry, we do not lose sight of the benefits social work services can offer home health care clients. Also, with the writing of this book, I hope to share with other agencies the importance of having a quality social work program.

Ruth Ann Goode

Chapter 1

Introduction to Home Health Care: A Historical Perspective

The following vignettes reflect typical home health care situations across the United States:

Vignette #1

Ms. B, age fifty-two, was referred to the agency for high-risk diabetes after several emergency room visits at a local hospital. She was then referred to the social worker for an assessment and for community resources. The social worker observed that Ms. B lives alone in a low-income subsidized building. Ms. B is also feeling depressed, lonely, and has a limited social support system. The social worker assesses Ms. B and refers her to (a) a home health care agency for an evaluation of her depression, (b) a community-based waiver program for personal care and homemaker services and meals, and (c) arranges for her to go to the zoo with a group of residents from her building. The goal is to empower her and reduce her isolation and improve her overall medical status. Ms. B is very pleased with her social work services.

Vignette #2

Mrs. J, age eighty-one, was recently discharged from the hospital. She lives alone in an apartment, is ambulatory, uses a walker, and needs some assistance in activities of daily living. On a routine visit by a home health agency nurse, Mrs. J expresses to the nurse that she needs help with meals and cleaning. The nurse tells her that she can call the local Office for the Aging and they will help her. The nurse leaves and Mrs. J forgets to call the agency. The home health agency has no social worker and the nurse does what she is expected to do.

Both cases are characteristic of home health agencies. It is also common for some home health agencies to employ social workers or offer social work services to their clients. In agencies that do not offer social work services, many home health clients do not receive adequate psychosocial or team-oriented care.

Home health care is a rather diverse and dynamic service industry. More than 20,000 agencies provide home care services to some eight million individuals who require services because of an acute illness, long-term health problems, disability, or terminal illness. Annual costs for home care were $40 billion in 1997 and are expected to exceed $42 billion in 1998 (National Association of Home Care, 1999).

Medicare's enactment in 1965 accelerated the growth of the industry. In 1973, these services were made available to the disabled. Between 1967 and 1985, the number of agencies grew from 1,753 to over 5,983. In the 1980s, the number of agencies leveled off at about 5,900 and now has actually decreased because of paperwork, unreliable payment policies, and the move toward prospective payment (National Association of Home Care, 1999).

Estimates show that as many as 9 million to 11 million Americans need home health care services. Most of the elderly population receive services from so-called informal caregivers—family members, friends, or others who provide uncompensated care. Some of this population receive formal services (i.e., purchased or compensated services from home health care providers) (National Association of Home Care, 1999). Reasons cited for this increased industry are many, including the increased graying of our population, increased long-term and health needs of the elderly population, changed consumer preference for home care, the adoption of sophisticated technology, and changed federal policy on deinstitutionalization. The diagnostic related groups (DRG) regulations for hospitals in the mid-1980s stimulated growth even more. Fewer agencies are losing money, and the industry has become extremely profitable (Health Care Financing Administration, 1992).

Home health care is the fastest-growing segment of the health service industry, and employment in home health care has doubled since 1988. The largest groups of employees include home health aides and registered nurses. Currently, approximately 7,000 social workers represent full-time equivalent employees. Many of these social workers also only work part time (as needed), or as independent contractors (National Association of Home Care, 1999). Upon completing my research, I found that many agencies are unable to employ enough social workers. Health care workers said they would expect higher utilization and more employment growth if agencies really understood the social work practice area and the benefits of having a program.

Home health care staff provide intermittent, skilled care visits to patients in their homes or natural environments. Medicare insists on a medically driven model, with nursing care being the focus. Nevertheless, Medicare does recognize the importance of allied services and the care is reimbursed. These services include physical therapy, speech therapy, occupational therapy, home health aide services, nutrition care, and medical social work services. Medicare reinforces a holistic approach to meeting medical, nursing, social, rehabilitative, psychological, and emotional needs of patients.

Medicare reimburses agencies for social work services and encourages a team-oriented approach to psychosocial care. In agencies that have social work staff, the social workers do psychosocial care, enabling the nurses to perform their tasks much more efficiently. Thus, these agencies bring in more revenue. When nurses have to perform both tasks, the agencies suffer in revenue and productivity.

The history of home health care is fascinating in that, traditionally, there are strong emphases on comprehensive psychosocial care for individuals and families. The Visiting Nurse Association (VNA) is the leader in this area.

The underlying policy that affects home health care services in the United States is very fragmented and is driven by funding mechanisms. Medicare, the major funding source, is medically oriented, requiring specific diagnosis and orders by a physician, and the service is on a short-term, intermittent visit basis. To date, the social worker's role is secondary and limited, and Medicare does not mandate that patients be assessed or followed up. The nurse, or case manager, and physician decide which patients to refer and which patients to discharge. When the patient's care medically closes, the social worker's responsibility also closes, often prematurely. This severely limits meeting the psychosocial needs of the patient. The National Association of Social Workers (NASW, 1991) formed a Home Health Care Task Force, conducted a study, and found three major problem areas:

1. Social work is not a skilled, independent, reimbursed service, and there are no mandatory guidelines, even though data suggest that social work intervention expedites treatment compliance and prevents rehospitalization.
2. There are no consistent state or regional guidelines. One regulatory agency in the study allowed and reimbursed limited visits, and another agency only allowed three to four visits. Therefore, patients living in one geographic area were receiving excellent psychosocial care and those in another area were neglected. The state and regional intermediaries contradicted Medicare rules.
3. Some regulatory agencies are reimbursing for assessment-only visits. Also, since Medicare expanded medical social work (MSW) services in July, 1989 to include counseling, it is not clear whether there has been an impact.

MEDICAL SOCIAL SERVICES

Medical social services have been an integral part of the provision of health service since 1905. In 1955, the U.S. Public Health Services endorsed a physician-oriented organized home health care team designed to provide medical and social services to patients within their homes. The team consisted of a physician, nurse, and social worker. Since 1965, Medicare has provided reimbursement for medical social work services in home health care equal to or greater than that for nursing. Medicare recognizes services that are needed for patients' total functioning. An interdisciplinary approach is necessary to aid patients in regaining their independence and highest level of functioning. Social workers assist patients and their families to adapt and plan their home environments. Social work services help relieve stress; provide crisis intervention; assist with financial problems; and provide advocacy, community services, information and referral, emotional support, appropriate counseling, and education. Even though social work is not recognized as a primary service, visits are reimbursed and, as of July 1, 1989, counseling visits are covered (NASW, 1991). Agencies are not required to provide social work services; they decide which ancillary services to offer.

What encourages or discourages agencies from providing social work services is not known. Are agencies afraid of nonreimbursement? Are there staff shortages? Are agencies knowledgeable about Medicare regulations? Are agencies aware of the revenue they are missing? Are nurses providing the services? These are questions I examine.

HOME HEALTH CARE SERVICES

The continuum of care for the homebound or semihomebound elderly in the community begins with services such as friendly visiting, meals-on-wheels (or volunteers to deliver meals), escort, chores, lifeline-type programs that provide a mechanical means of communication with service providers or emergency response systems, daily friendly telephone calls, and daily personal checks by the Postal Service.

Mid-range home health care services are provided by semiprofessional personnel, including home attendants, homemakers, home health aides, and personal care assistants. These individuals' responsibilities range from purely household support functions, such as meal preparation, shopping, laundry, and cleaning, to personal care and hands-on functions, such as assistance with grooming, dressing, toileting, and eating, to social-therapeutic forms of help, such as supportive companionship. Traditionally, designated ancillary or supplemental services are frequently combined to form the central core of the home health care agency's available array of services.

Home health care entails the delivery of an expanding array of more traditional professional service functions, including, more frequently, visiting nurse services and home visits by local social workers and, less frequently, periodic assistance from recreational therapists, occupational therapists, physical therapists, dentists, physicians, psychiatrists, speech and language pathologists, nutritionists, psychologists, legal specialists, and clergy (Kaye, 1992).

Most often, the missing ingredient is case management or service coordination. This function is usually performed by a medical social worker, if an agency offers the service. Home health care, by definition, assumes a more sophisticated repertoire of services than any single intervention described above. Because home health care is more often than not only part of a service package, case management becomes a particularly important ingredient (Kaye, 1992). Often, social workers are needed to assume this role.

Currently the most sophisticated and comprehensive form of home health care available is probably long-term home health care programs. These programs offer, in addition to a home health aide or home attendant, regular nursing service, social service, meals-on-wheels, and, when necessary, physical therapists; all are part of the basic service package. Naturally, the case management role is explicit under such circumstances and often includes the overseeing of services other than those provided by the home health care agency itself. Information and referral services may be standard components of long-term home health care.

APPROPRIATE CLIENTS AND THEIR PROBLEMS

The range of potential home health care service recipients is large and diverse. It encompasses the developmentally disabled, post-hospitalization patients, the disabled and chronically impaired of all ages, the mentally ill, the terminally ill requiring hospice care at home, newborn infants and their mothers, and abused children and older adults.

Home health care has a long tradition of responding to the needs of older adults. Many argue, however, that the aged, by virtue of the extended period of time in which they have lived, represent a particularly heterogeneous group, presenting a seemingly endless variety of needs and requests for support. This diversity dictates the importance of establishing a wide range of flexible interventions and programs in the home health care situation.

Many situations, both personal and environmental, require the initiation of home health care services for older adults. The presence of one or more of these risk factors dramatically increases the likelihood that home health care is needed. Health care professionals involved in the referral process need to keep an especially keen eye on elderly adults in the community who have any of the following risk factors.

Acute Disability

Unexpected accidents such as falls and acute illnesses signal the need for time-limited home health care assistance. Services are needed only as long as the healing process is underway or recovery progresses.

Chronic Disability

Long-term impairment due to chronic illness or disease (e.g., stroke, heart disease, arthritis) is an all-too-common factor instigating the need for services. Frequently, services are needed for an extended period in such cases.

Absence or Lack of Social Supports

Although the majority of community care for the elderly continues to be provided by the family unit, it is not unusual for individuals age seventy and older to outlive a large segment of their natural support networks, including family, friends, and neighbors. If significant others are not outlived, they may have their own problems to grapple with, leaving them unavailable to care for the elderly. Weak or nonexistent support networks place the impaired older person in severe jeopardy.

Impaired Ability to Handle Activities of Daily Living

The functional and physical activities of daily living (ADL) must be performed if an individual is to continue living in the community with any degree of dignity or quality of life. The inability to accomplish one or more basic activities of daily living is a prime measure of the need for outside assistance.

Psychological or Cognitive Decline

Periods of mental confusion or disorientation place the older adult residing in the community at high risk. Such individuals may become a danger to themselves and to others. Home health care serves as an effective intervention when the condition is episodic, whereby intermittent assistance is adequate.

The Experience of a Traumatic Event

It is not unusual for a sudden, highly stressful event to exacerbate impairing conditions in the elderly. The death of a spouse, sudden alterations in the environment, temporary or permanent loss of autonomy, relocation of a close friend, and a robbery or mugging can cause a downturn in physical or mental health and bring about a need for outside help.

Depending on the nature of the precipitating factors, home health care assumes rehabilitative, custodial, and maintenance assistance, or a combination of these functions.

HOME HEALTH ORGANIZATIONS

Home health care services are provided by any number of organizational sources, including public programs, vendor programs, private or nonprofit groups, and proprietary or for-profit organizations. Similarly, home health care may be freestanding, that is, the exclusive program offered by an agency, or it may be one of many services offered by a facility or company.

More and more hospitals and long-term care facilities are offering home health care services, which means that health-related and skilled nursing care, hospital services, and apartments for the aged make up the total service package. Similarly, an increasing number of national home health care companies offer not only home-based services, but are in the business of selling and renting durable medical equipment and health products as well. Home health care services may be relatively small ancillary programs attached to large organizations, such as home health care programs housed within large-scale hospitals and medical centers. In the case of private auspice home health care programs, services are frequently third party and reimbursable by Medicare, Medicaid, private insurance policies, Blue Cross/Blue Shield, health maintenance organizations (HMOs), and group health plans.

Funding for home health care is provided by at least five federal programs. Medically oriented home health care is funded through Titles XVIII and XIX of the Social Security Act. On the other hand, programs that emphasize social and personal care services are supported through Title XX of the Social Security Act and Title III of the Older Americans Act. In addition, the Veterans Administration provides funding for both social and health-related home health care services. Of course, a substantial portion of home health care is financed through private and commercial insurance companies, charitable and philanthropic groups, and out-of-pocket expenditures by the elderly and their families (Kaye, 1992).

With third-party payments, clients are covered by Medicaid or Medicare for services received. This type of payment is determined by a variety of factors, including client diagnosis, the types of services required, the category of personnel providing care, and the circumstances under which assistance is needed, such as hours of services offered per day or week. Certain services and periods of coverage are not reimbursable. Furthermore, certain agencies are not reimbursable under Medicaid or Medicare because they are uncertified. The types of coverage available through major legislative mechanisms mandating home health care should be examined.

MEDICARE

Medicare coverage of home health care is authorized by Title XVII of the Social Security Act. Either Part A (Hospital Insurance) or Part B (Medical Insurance) pays for services. Eligibility criteria center on the need for intermittent skilled nursing, physical therapy, or speech therapy. Confinement to one's home, or homebound status, is required, along with a physician's certification of need and establishment of a home health care plan. There are no time constraints for coverage, such as limitations on the maximum number of allowable visits, and no requirement for prior hospitalization, as long as all conditions of eligibility are satisfied. The client must require skilled care.

Medical coverage is not available for clients who are solely in need of custodial or maintenance care; assistance in performing the activities of daily living, such as household services, shopping, and meal preparation; assistance with bathing and dressing; or medical social work services. Homemaker services are not eligible for coverage. Medicare continues to pay for home health visits as long as skilled nursing, physical therapy, or speech therapy are involved.

Funding for Medicare home health services is open ended; that is, there is no cap on the amount expended, but utilization patterns reflect low levels of expenditure. Reimbursed home health care services must be provided by a certified home health agency. In regional areas, Medicare reimburses certified home health agencies in a manner similar to that of hospitals; insurance companies and similar fiscal intermediaries assist in the administration of the program by processing claims, determining eligibility, and reimbursing reasonable costs. Health care professionals have particularly strong responsibility for obtaining well-documented evidence concerning clients' eligibility and care.

Medicare does not cover such services as full-time nursing care at home, drugs and biologicals, home-delivered meals, blood transfusions and, as mentioned earlier, homemaker services (Kaye, 1992).

Medicare recipients are the largest group of clients needing home health care services. This group of the elderly are at risk and often do not have access to social work services. Medicare reimburses home health agencies for social work visits, but it is not known what variables affect utilization.

Services Covered by Medicare

1. Observation and assessment of client's condition when only the specialized skills of a medical professional can determine a client's status
2. Management and evaluation of a client care plan
3. Teaching and training activities
4. Administration of medications
5. Tube feedings
6. Nasopharyngeal and tracheotomy aspiration
7. Catheters
8. Wound care
9. Ostomy care
10. Heart treatments
11. Medical gases
12. Rehabilitation nursing
13. Venipuncture
14. Student nurse visits
15. Psychiatric evaluation and therapy (Health Care Financing Administration, 1992)

Hospice Care

In 1983, Medicare expanded and began to include coverage of in-home hospice care. Individuals with terminal illnesses now receive a comprehensive set of medical and support services. The mission of hospice care is to provide noncurative care to the terminally ill; only pain-relieving medications and treatments are offered. The underlying philosophy includes the patient's right to death and dignity in familiar surroundings of family, friends, and cherished possessions. Hospice services are offered by hospitals, home health care agencies, nursing homes, or community-based organizations. Care must be provided by a Medicare-certified hospice if coverage is to be approved. Covered services include physician services; nursing services; medical appliances; supplies and outpatient drugs for symptom management and pain relief; home health aide and homemaker services; physical, occupational, and speech therapies; medical social services; counseling; and short-term, inpatient respite care. Whereas home health care under Medicare covers an unlimited number of home visits, hospice care extends its services for two periods of ninety days each and one period of thirty days, plus an optional permanent extension under the condition that the patient remains terminally ill. Part A and Part B of Medicare reimburse for hospice services.

MEDICAID

As a rule, Title XIX regulations stipulate a fifty-fifty federal and state match. Elderly home health care recipients may be eligible for both Medicare and Medicaid. In such cases, Medicaid pays for Medicare premiums and deductibles. Medicaid also covers the cost of medical expenses delivered in the home that are not covered by Medicare, but that are included in a particular state's Medicaid program.

Medicaid does not reimburse for social work services provided by home health care agencies unless the client is enrolled in a waiver program to reduce nursing home stays. Ohio has such a program, called PASSPORT (Pre-Admission Screening and Services Program and Optimal Resources). Clients who are considered high risk for placement are provided case management by social workers, meals-on-wheels, homemaker services, personal care, respite care, transportation, day care, chores, and numerous other services. Clients such as the middle-income group, who have financial resources, are not eligible for Medicaid.

Chapter 2

The Utilization of Social Work Services in Twelve Home Health Care Agencies: A Research Study

PURPOSE

This research study, conducted in 1995, explores health care professionals' attitudes and beliefs about social work services and who should provide psychosocial care. An emphasis is placed on gaining insight into the utilization of social work services and on what enhances or hinders this provision of care.

This study specifically focuses on the attitudes, beliefs, and perceptions of nurses, administrative staff, and physical and occupational therapists pertaining to social work services. The results show that under Medicare, independent, skilled providers decide whether clients need social work services; therefore, they directly affect service delivery. This study also examines regulatory guidelines in the states of Michigan, Ohio, Illinois, Indiana, and Wisconsin.

Significance

The study is significant in that it contributes to both the nursing and social work professions. It provides insight into the team approach to patient care and how team members contribute to patient care and to each other.

An interdisciplinary team approach is necessary to (1) treat the patient-family system; (2) relieve stress; (3) provide crisis intervention, financial assistance, advocacy, and supportive counseling; and (4) assist in making long-term care plans. Social work services can prevent unnecessary hospital stays, costly medical bills, and improve compliance. In addition, social workers are important links to community resources. This study provides insight into how nursing staff and social workers together facilitate holistic patient care.

Relationship of the Study to Changes in the Social Work Profession

With changes in the structuring, financing, and philosophy of health care delivery, patients are being discharged from hospitals early, often more debilitated and at great risk. Due to the fact that families and caregivers continue to have more responsibility on a twenty-four-hour basis, family life is becoming disrupted. Roles change, relationships become strained, financial problems occur, and families do not know where to turn for help. With an ever-increasing aging population, cost-containment efforts, and increasing high technology, home health care continues to grow. Social and emotional rehabilitation continue to be recognized as critical tasks of the health care team. Social workers in home health care strive to improve and maintain social, emotional, environmental, functional, physical, and mental health needs of patients and families. Social workers coordinate care and bridge the gap between acute care and long-term care.

METHODOLOGY

This study explores and describes home health care providers' attitudes and perceptions of social work services and who should provide psychosocial care. Because of the emphasis on understanding social and psychological phenomena, the methodology selected was qualitative, using an emergent, discovery, and theory-building design known as grounded theory (Glaser and Strauss, 1967). The overall methodology was inductive, using unstructured interviews and participant observation with content analysis. There was a purposive sampling of twelve home health care agencies and a case study method was used to report data collected.

This chapter describes the details of the research design utilized, assumptions prior to the study, research questions, and procedures used in the study. It includes a description of the methodology used for data collection and data analysis, a discussion of the scope and limitations of this study, and major findings and conclusions.

Nature of the Study

An unstructured, open-ended interview was the instrument used to collect data. The investigator developed a topical outline to elicit respondents' feelings, beliefs, experiences, and attitudes. The investigator feels that this provides more related inquiry into team-oriented patient care and encourages discovery, insight, and theory emergence. This design also allows for the collection of demographic data related to the agencies that participated in the study.

Grounded theory is a highly systematic research approach for the collection and analysis of qualitative data for the purpose of generating explanatory theory that gives further understanding of social and psychological phenomena. The purpose of grounded theory is to develop theory that explains basic patterns or interactions that occur in social life (Chenitz and Swanson, 1986). Grounded theory has its roots in the social sciences and is used in qualitative studies in the disciplines of sociology, psychology, and social work. It also has gained more popularity in the nursing field.

The grounded theory approach is useful in conceptualizing human behavior and interactions within complex situations, and is especially useful in understanding emerging social problems. Above all, grounded theory makes its greatest contribution in areas where little research has been done. Therefore, one of the major uses of grounded theory is in preliminary, exploratory, and descriptive studies (Glaser and Strauss, 1967). The specific focus is to generate a theory that can be used as a precursor for other research. The approach uses a constant comparison technique whereby interviews and field notes are continuously compared until a pattern or theory emerges. Data collection continues until categories and relationships become saturated and no new data or additions are made. One or more overriding theories or concepts will emerge.

With grounded theory, an intensive or qualitative interview is the best vehicle for eliciting personal and private concerns. The inductive design of the grounded theory study adheres to the following sequence:

**Design study → collect data → analyze data →
develop hypotheses → develop theory**

The study consisted of major research questions that guided the inquiry and content analyses. Because the study was exploratory in nature and there was a need to study health care professionals' attitudes and perceptions about social workers, the grounded theory approach was most appropriate.

Assumptions

Home health agencies should provide holistic, team-oriented, coordinated care. An interdisciplinary approach is needed to treat the patient-family system in the context of its social environment. Social work services should be provided by a social worker with an MSW degree and two years of health care experience, or at least a BSW with MSW supervision. Social work services should be provided by Medicare-certified agencies and the social work staff should be available at all times.

RESEARCH QUESTIONS

The following research questions are appropriate in an exploratory, grounded theory study:

1. Do home health care agencies currently have a policy on who provides psychosocial care?
2. How will different types of agencies respond and what trends are developing?
3. What are the hindrances to providing social work services in this context?
4. Who provides psychosocial care at this time?
5. Are agencies aware of revenue possibilities from providing social work services?

To gain knowledge related to these major research questions, the open-ended interview topic summary should be as follows:

- Agency, location.
- Names and positions of interviewees.
- Type of agency, case mix.
- Number of employees, contract staff.
- Approximate number of total home health care visits.
- Does your agency provide social work services?
- If not, what have you found to be the obstacles to providing social work services?
- How do you provide linkage to community resources?
- How involved are your nurses in providing psychosocial care?
- Do you feel your agency understands the Medicare standards for social work service?
- Has your agency ever received training in this area?
- Do you feel there is an adequate number of social workers working in or qualified to do home health care?
- What type of activities do you feel social workers should perform in home health care?

• Do you feel the Medicare standards need to be changed? How?
• Suggestions and comments.

PROCEDURES

The population for this study consisted of a purposive sample of twelve Medicare-certified home health agencies in the northeastern and central regions of Ohio. Recruitment letters were mailed to 100 home health agencies—taken from a list provided by Ohio Council of Home Health Care—requesting their voluntary participation in the study. Twelve agencies were selected based on their size, location, and regulatory involvement. After the final proposal was approved, the investigator relocated to Cleveland, so most of the agencies were located in that area. In addition, the investigator wanted a purposive sample of rural, urban, and suburban agencies. Also, it was important to have four for-profit agencies, four non-profit agencies, and four hospital-based agencies.

Because of the emphasis on discovery and theory building, the tools for data gathering included an open-ended, unstructured interview at each agency with the administrator or director, the director of nursing, and a separate focus group interview of clinical staff. The focus group within each agency consisted of eight to ten home health care professionals, including physical therapists, occupational therapists, home health aides, and RN case managers.

The interviews and focus groups were conducted by the investigator using brief general outlines of major topics and themes. A consent form was signed by each participant, and each interview and focus group lasted about one and a half hours. The interviews were audiotaped and then summarized into field notes. The interviews and focus groups were held in a large conference room, with coffee and a round table setup to encourage more related natural inquiry. A sample recruitment letter, focus group questions, and consent forms are exhibited in Appendixes A, B, and C.

Data Analysis

Each interview was audiotaped and labeled. The investigator transcribed the tapes into field notes and analyzed each tape using the grounded theory approach of Glaser and Strauss (1967). This approach included discovering trends and categories of findings, linking trends, identifying care categories, and refining the theory. Secondary data analysis included the review and summary of agency job descriptions, agency brochures, social work utilization statistics, home health care visits, philosophies, policies, and procedures. Responses to open-ended questions were summarized into trends and each agency was analyzed from a case study method and multisite analysis.

SCOPE AND LIMITATIONS

The goal of social work service in home health care is to improve or maintain the social, emotional, functional, and physical health status of the patient, as well as to enhance the coping skills of the family or caregiver system. The underlying approach is based on the medical model, which consists of a medical diagnosis, a physician's order, and only episodic, short-term visits by registered nurses. Usually, there is a limit of thirty-eight to sixty days of intermittent visits. This is a major limitation and is one of the reasons why home health care agencies do not offer social work services. Furthermore, the social worker has to be well versed in Medicare regulations to assure reimbursement for the agency. For this reason, this study was limited only to Medicare-certified agencies. Medicare is the only program that reimburses for social work services.

This study was limited to northeastern and central Ohio. The results hold potential to be generalized to apply to other regions, including areas in Illinois, Michigan, and Indiana. The Medicare intermediaries or regulatory agencies that control Ohio's agencies are in these states. Furthermore, field or interview research has some intrinsic limitations. The conclusions drawn from qualitative interview research are often regarded as suggestive rather than definitive.

Subjectivity could have been a limiting factor because the researcher's orientation might have affected results. Some of the agencies knew the researcher professionally and may have been more honest and open because of that relationship. The use of purposive sampling is in itself a less generalized method. However, in this study this approach was necessary in order to gain permission to conduct the research.

Because research pertaining to the social worker's role in Medicare-certified agencies in these selected states had not been systematically done, this study provided an initial entry into this topic. Moreover, the researcher feels the study was worthwhile and was a sound exploratory experience.

FINDINGS AND ANALYSIS

This section presents findings from the research and provides an analysis relative to the literature review. First, the findings from the multisite care analysis are described in several major theoretical clusters and factors resulting from the study. These clusters include roles and responsibilities of home health care social workers, referrals and utilization, understanding of Medicare standards for home health care, staff recruitment, retention and training, obstacles in providing social work services, community service needs, staffing trends, policy issues, reimbursement issues, future plans for the social work program, and agency auspice or structure. Second, these findings and their relationship to the literature review are analyzed. Major areas of literature review include home health services with the elderly, medical social work and discharge planning, interdisciplinary team practice, policy issues, Medicare standards, health care in the future, social work practices in home health care, health care reform, group work, and bioethical issues. Literature review gaps are also addressed.

Summary of Findings

Roles and Responsibilities of Social Workers

All twelve home health care agencies gave the same responses regarding the responsibilities of social workers in home health care. Social workers' tasks include psychosocial assessments, working with poor family dynamics, community resource linkages, assisting families with financial problems, long-term planning, and placements. Five agencies also felt social workers were helpful in the assessment of safety and risk factors of patients. One agency even utilized a part-time bachelor's level social worker in its billing department to determine appropriate payer sources and assist patients in applying for benefits to which they were entitled.

Referrals and Utilization

Eleven of the twelve agencies had social work programs and eagerly made patient referrals. One agency did not provide social work services because it had limited knowledge and no available staff. Seven indicated that their social work programs were recently developed within the past year and were still in transition. All eleven agencies indicated that their overall utilization increased as they added social work staff. These agencies also indicated that their social work staff must be available to see patients in a timely manner or the utilization and visits decreased. Thus, availability became a key factor.

Medicare Standards for Social Work Practice

All twelve agencies indicated they had very little knowledge of Medicare standards and rules related to the provision of social work services. All agencies reported a serious need for education and systematic knowledge.

Only one agency knew that Medicare does not reimburse for visits to do Medicaid applications for patients. Two thought that their Medicare intermediaries only allowed two to four social work visits per patient. Five agencies indicated they left it up to their social workers, hoping there would be no denials. Four indicated they had no idea about the subject of allowed visits. None of the twelve knew that Medicare passed an amendment in 1989 allowing counseling visits if they related to medical conditions of patients, and that Medicare had no limit on visits as long as the worker justified "skilled" status. All twelve agencies reported they had no knowledge of what constituted a skilled social work visit. Only two agencies knew that Medicare also reimbursed for an assessment visit on each patient, which they carried out. None of the twelve agencies knew that written materials were available from the National Association of Social Workers about guidelines and documentation.

Self-Recruitment, Retention, and Training

Staffing was a major concern for all twelve agencies. They indicated that home health care does not seem to attract social workers. They all reported that home health care requires a high level of independence, judgment, and credentials. Medicare standards require a master's level social worker or a bachelor's level social worker supervised by a master's level social worker. Seven agencies reported that recruiting experienced, independent social workers was very difficult. Retention was not a major problem because all of the agencies had new programs with new personnel. All twelve agencies reported a serious need for schools of social work to train more social workers in home health care and to use agencies as field training sites. Only one agency had trained students.

Obstacles to Providing Social Work Services

Obstacles to providing social work services consisted of three major areas: lack of knowledge on the part of physicians and the public about the benefits of social workers—reported by five agencies; lack of knowledge among the agencies—reported by ten agencies; and no reimbursement for social work visits, which prevented many patients from obtaining services—reported by all twelve agencies.

Community Service Gaps

All twelve home health care agencies indicated the same trends in community services needed to assist their patients on a long-term basis. These service gaps included transportation, meals-on-wheels, available nursing home beds, respite care, day care, PASSPORT services, chore services, and financial assistance.

Two agencies indicated that they referred all of their patients to a social worker for a one-time assessment and that the social worker determined the need for future visits. One agency made limited referrals to an area office on aging because it did not have its own social work program. The remaining nine agencies left the screening to their nurses, who referred the patients to social workers.

The following factors were considered: high risks, safety concerns, need for long-term care, lack of support, inadequate living environment, family problems, financial problems, and need for community services. None of the agencies were aware of a formalized, written screening tool that was made available in 1992 by the National Association of Social Workers, "Screening Patients for Social Work Intervention."

Staffing Trends

In looking at the agencies, several staffing patterns emerged. Seven agencies employed their own social work staff and each one had a different constellation. One had a full-time MSW with two prn (as needed) social workers. One had two full-time MSWs; one had two part-time BSWs with MSW supervision. Another one had a full-time MSW with three prn social workers by contract. Another agency had two part-time MSWs; another one had one full-time BSW with MSW supervision, and another one had a full-time MSW. Four agencies contracted with MSW social workers for their staffing needs. Three out of four agencies had at least two contracts, but stated they primarily utilized a particular MSW who was experienced and more available. The fourth one contracted with an outside mental health agency for staffing. One agency had no social work program. The employment of social workers rather than contracting appeared to be the trend. Availability was also a key factor.

Policy Issues

All twelve agencies indicated that the fact that Medicaid does not reimburse for social work services was a major policy issue. Another major issue was that social work is secondary to nursing or physical therapy and services must be terminated when one of these disciplines discharges the patient. Six agencies indicated this as an issue and that social work should be an independent skilled service.

Reimbursement Issues

None of the agencies reported having a good working knowledge of reimbursement issues with social work. It was quite surprising that only one agency actually realized that social work produced significant revenue for its bottom line. Also, nine of the agencies were missing out on revenue because they were not aware that they could be doing more visits. Seven agencies reported a strong need for consultation on this issue.

Future Plans for Social Work Programs

Eleven agencies indicated that they planned to expand their existing social work programs, add staff, increase referrals, and extend their knowledge base about social work. One agency was interested in developing a program but needed outside consultation to do so.

Agency Auspice

The provision of social work service was not related to agency auspice. There were no differences in the proprietary, hospital-affiliated, or nonprofit agencies. The investigator expected to find stronger social work utilization among the nonprofit agencies. This did not appear to be demonstrated in this study.

Analysis of Findings in Relation to Literature Review

After an extensive review of the literature, it became apparent that this study focused on a very specific area that had not been thoroughly or systematically investigated. To date, there appears to be little research that deals with the way home health care staff treat social workers. Factors affecting home health care agency utilization of social work services appear to be a major area of inquiry missing in earlier published research.

The data in this study support several segments of the literature, including home health care services to the elderly, social work and discharge planning, health care and future directions, interdisciplinary teams, policy issues, Medicare standards, health care reform, and social work practice in home health care. The study negates two major areas of the literature: group work and bioethical practice. Some differences on team issues will also be addressed.

Home Health Care Services for the Elderly

The first cluster of literature focuses on home health care services delivered to the elderly. The aging of America is a trend that places serious strains on our health care system. The demand for nursing homes is soaring. The elderly are the heaviest users of health care. They make up 12 percent of the population, but they account for almost 40 percent of all hospital admissions, 20 percent of physician visits, and almost 50 percent of the prescription drug market. Health care for the elderly presents an array of issues, such as cost effectiveness, allocation of resources, methods of insurance, and establishment of priorities for research and service delivery. All of the agencies reported that their caseloads consisted primarily of the geriatric population.

Medicare began to influence medical social work in the 1960s. New areas of practice for the elderly began to emerge at that time, including casework and counseling, financial planning and assistance, consultation with physicians, liaison with the community, education and research, outpatient care, home health, and nursing homes. Medicare reimbursement strategies began to develop (Watts, 1967).

Wattenberg and McGann (1984) stress the need for community-based and hospital social workers to assist older patients in completing insurance forms and applications for programs of entitlement, such as Medicare, Medicaid, food stamps, discounts, and other programs.

This study substantiates the importance these areas of social work practice. All of the agencies reported the roles and responsibilities of social workers as being the same areas that have been influenced by Medicare coverage.

Medical Social Work and Discharge Planning

The second literature cluster focuses on medical social work and discharge planning. In the literature on discharge planning and advocacy there are three broad categories, each of which reflects the knowledge base needed for practicing social workers. The three categories are: (1) the role and appropriateness of discharge planning and advocacy as a function of professional social work, (2) skills and knowledge required for the practice of discharge planning and advocacy, and (3) evaluation and demonstration of discharge models and approaches.

Discharge planning is inextricably tied to developing resources for the posthospital care of the patient (Lurie, Pinskey, and Tuzman, 1981). Sandman (1981) identifies five stages in the discharge planning process: (1) assessment, (2) diagnosis, (3) prescription, (4) implementation, and (5) evaluation. The role of the social worker is to explain and manage the psychosocial elements of patient care, specifically as they relate to discharge planning. The same stages were reported in this study. Home health care agencies have also taken on a discharge planning process.

Another important component of discharge planning is helping patients plan for their future needs at a time of stress and crises. Many patients do not plan for crises and therefore are unprepared for posthospitalization contingencies. This is particularly true for elderly patients who do not have adequate support systems, such as family or friends, to accommodate them following hospitalization (Coulton et al., 1982). Other factors that interfere with successful posthospital care are lack of adequate resources such as extended-care beds, limited cooperation of medical staff in preparing necessary paperwork, and the changing medical condition of the patient (Lurie, Pinskey, and Tuzman, 1981; Schrager et al., 1978). Social workers have a traditional role to work directly with patients and to develop and advocate programs that ensure access to high-quality care at all times (Coulton et al., 1982; Lurie, Pinskey, and Tuzman, 1981).

In this study, long-term planning was reported as a major social work task, and post-home health care resources were cited as a problem due to service gaps.

Interdisciplinary Team Practice

The literature reviewed in this cluster discusses issues such as team development (Lee, 1980), the administrative support and structure needed to create and use an interdisciplinary team conference (Clarke, Distasi, and Wallace, 1978), and interagency collaboration for health planning.

This study very strongly supports team practice. Interdisciplinary team conferences were reported as crucial in promoting the social work staff as team players. Team conferences also promote higher utilization of services.

Other research focuses on themes, such as professional identity, role overlap and conflict (Lowe and Herranen, 1978), boundaries and areas of professional expertise, the team as reflective of systemic and patient care problems, and ethical issues and decision making (Abramson, 1984).

Ben-Sira and Szyf (1992) conducted a demonstration study among thirty-four social worker/nurse teams who worked on the same hospital ward in Israel. The study aimed to elucidate the conditions for promoting a milieu of collaboration between nurses and social workers. The data suggested that this collaboration was characterized by status inequality, with the nurses' dominance prevailing with respect to meeting the patients' psychosocial needs. Nurses viewed social workers mainly as performing chores related to the patients' instrumental needs outside the hospital, while social workers, though overtly objecting to the nurses' dominance, still viewed the milieu as collaborative.

Explanations were offered for this apparent contradiction. Possible implications were suggested regarding the consequences for effectively meeting the psychosocial needs of patients and for the professional status of social workers in hospitals.

This study does not appear to support this phenomenon. Although nursing was dominant in home health care, social workers did not report inequality and nurses did not regard social workers as fulfilling chores. Teamwork and collaboration were important. Most of these data were obtained from hospitals rather than home health care. Very few studies have been done on role conflict in home health care.

Policy Issues

Another literature segment involved policy issues. Policies affect social work services in home health care practice (NASW, 1991). Since the introduction of Medicare in the 1960s, home health care services have become structured around a medical model, or a hospital service on wheels (Olson and Mintun, 1990). As a result, home health care has lost much of its human services or family and community approach.

This study also supports the medical model concept and a reimbursement-driven system. Home health care has become more of a business.

The availability of funding to support social work services, education, and research depends on decisions made in the public policy realm (Kane, 1985). Evidence was reported in the study regarding lack of funding for low-income patients or those on Medicaid.

Medicare Standards for Social Work Practice
in Home Health Care

Another large segment of literature relates to Medicare standards for social workers in home health care. To date, the role of social workers in home health care in the United States is secondary. Medicare's conditions of participation for home health agencies mandate that social work services be available to patients, but do not require that patients be seen by social workers or that social workers be involved in the design of the care plan or subsequent assessments. A nurse usually decides whether social work intervention is needed. This study substantiates the literature. Social work continues to play a secondary role and an assessment is not mandatory.

The medical emphasis of Medicare and Medicaid programs ignores the fact that many of the problems and needs of home health care recipients are complex, extending beyond the purely medical sphere. This is particularly true of elderly people, who are the majority of home health care patients and whose frailties and limitations often result from social and mental deficits as well as from physical impairments (NASW, 1991).

The National Association of Social Workers (NASW, 1991) has issued the following policy statement:

> Resolving the identified problems that interfere with the effective provision of home health care, social work services will serve to support patients and their caregiver systems who wish to continue health care in the home. Resolving the problems will also promote the cost-effective provision of home health care.

The National Association of Social Workers recommends that these problems be resolved by:

- granting skilled status to medical social work services under Medicare, thus establishing social work intervention as a qualifying service in home health;
- specifying a clear and uniform delineation of home health social work services that are reimbursable under Medicare;

- recognizing assessment and follow-up service, including case management by a home health social worker, as a skilled, reimbursable service under Medicare;
- recognizing medical social work services as a reimbursable benefit under Medicaid;
- monitoring implementation of the July 1990 amendment to Medicare, part B, and advancing professional autonomy for home health care social workers. (p. 2)

The impact of this new policy is not known. In 1991, NASW noted the following:

Data suggest that early social work assessment and intervention in home health care expedite shorter periods of nursing and other medical services. This study appeared to substantiate that these major issues were not yet resolved. (p. 5)

Health Care in the Future

Griff and Lerman (1987) also predict that high-tech home health care will be a rapidly growing area. The development of sophisticated technologies—such as home intravenous antibiotic therapy, total parenteral nutrition therapy, cancer chemotherapy, and tracheotomy care—facilitates early hospital discharge and increases the number of treatments that can be given in the home. High-technology home therapy is one of the most rapidly growing segments of the home health care field, and is expected to transform the home into the primary site of clinical care in the twenty-first century (Griff and Lerman, 1987). All of the agencies reported doing high-tech home health care, and this type of care is expected to continue to expand.

Social Work Practice Areas

The literature review demonstrates that the social worker in home health care is uniquely qualified to perform five major areas of practice with patients and their families: (1) assessment of social and emotional factors; (2) counseling for long-range planning and decision making; (3) community resources and linkage; (4) short-term therapy; and (5) intervention for high-risk patients. High-risk areas include abuse, neglect, inadequate food or supplies, and potential suicide (Health Care Financing Administration, 1990). As of July 1, 1989, social workers provide counseling for adjustment to illness and there is no limit on visits, as long as there is appropriate documentation. Also, social workers evaluate safety and environmental factors of patients living alone, who need additional services.

Patients' problems fall into four major areas that require intervention: (1) counseling and support for adjustment to illness; (2) living arrangements, such as inadequate housing; (3) financial problems; and (4) the need for services (Goode, 1992). Home health care involves care in the client's place of residence; however, the residence or living arrangement at times is one of the major factors contributing to the client's health problems. All of the agencies in the study agreed on the roles and responsibilities of social workers but had little or no knowledge of the 1989 standard on counseling visits.

Health Care Reform

Another segment of literature involves health care reform. The United States must solve at least three problems that have been dealt with by other major industrialized countries: (1) the poor and disadvantaged must be provided with health services, health insurance, or the financial means to purchase health insurance; (2) for the nonpoor, a mechanism must be found to pool health risks while reforming private health insurance (e.g., having guaranteed issues, eliminating preexisting conditions, and nonrenewability clauses); and (3) mechanisms must be found to control costs (Health Care Financing Administration, 1992). These problems also were substantiated in the study.

Group Work by Social Workers

Group work has become a significant mode of social work intervention in health care settings and is reviewed in the literature. Much of this literature describes groups or group programs for patients and families who are coping with the psychological effects of a particular disease or life crisis, such as aging or institutionalization. Most of the literature includes a discussion of the special needs of the given population, the rationale for using a group approach, and the format or structure of the group. This was not demonstrated in the study because none of the agencies had groups.

Bioethical Issues

Another cluster focuses on bioethical issues in social work practice. Bernstein (1980) outlines legal principles and issues commonly facing social workers. This valuable review examines the right to a natural death, anatomical gifts, power of attorney, joint bank accounts, wills, insurance, and estates. The social worker plays an important role when such legal issues arise, by providing useful information and referrals, as well as by helping the patient and family cope with complex issues at a time of stress.

Gelman (1986) considers decisions involving prolongation of life and the participation of the social worker in those decisions. Both Gelman (1986) and Reamer (1985) advocate the establishment of a hospital ethics committee on which the social worker plays an active role. The social worker who understands the dynamics of a life-and-death situation can support the patient and family. It is interesting that only one agency mentioned these issues in the present study, and none of the agencies had ethics committees. It was predicted that change would eventually occur.

CONCLUSIONS AND IMPLICATIONS
FOR FUTURE APPLICATIONS AND RESEARCH

The objective of this study was to explore the attitudes, perceptions, and beliefs of home health care staff about social workers and how they may affect the utilization of social work services.

This section summarizes the findings and conclusions from this research study and how they relate to future applications and research. These findings apply to four major areas: (1) social work practice in home health care, (2) home health care providers, (3) social work education, and (4) policy issues. The section concludes with implications for future research.

Eight major conclusions were drawn from common themes in responses from all twelve agencies. The first area relates to tasks and responsibilities of social workers in home health care. All of the agencies had a good working knowledge of what home health care social workers do with patients and families. Two major roles include doing psychosocial assessments and community resource linkages.

The second area relates to factors affecting referrals and utilization of services. Utilization of social work services is directly linked to three major factors: (1) staffing and availability, (2) knowledge of the benefits that social work offers, and (3) treatment of social work staff as team players. Overall, referrals tend to increase if there are available staff, if the clinical staff have good knowledge of what social workers do to benefit patients and families, and if agencies hold regular team-oriented conferences to promote interaction among staff.

The third area relates to future development. All twelve agencies indicated that their social work programs were less than two years old and all expected referrals and staffing to increase in the future. One agency was beginning to develop a social work program and eleven agencies had existing programs.

The fourth area relates to Medicare standards and regulations and the degree of knowledge among home health care agency staff. All twelve agencies indicated they had very little knowledge of Medicare standards and rules related to the provision of social work services. All reported a serious need for education and systematic knowledge about Medicare standards. This prevented the agencies from providing good utilization of social work services.

The fifth area relates to staffing, recruitment, and training. Agencies reported they achieved better utilization of services by employing social workers rather than contracting with them. Also, all of the agencies reported that home health care does not seem to attract social workers. Seven agencies reported that recruiting experienced, independent, and knowledgeable social workers was very difficult. All twelve agencies reported a serious need for social work schools to train and expose students to home health care.

The sixth area relates to community service needs for patients. All of the agencies reported lack of services in several areas where their patients needed service after home health services were no longer required. These long-term services included transportation, meals-on-wheels, nursing home beds, respite care, day care, PASSPORT waiver services, chore services, and financial assistance.

The seventh area relates to obstacles in providing social work services. Agencies reported three major obstacles: (1) lack of knowledge about social workers on the part of physicians and the public; (2) lack of knowledge among home health care agencies; and (3) lack of reimbursement by Medicaid.

The eighth area relates to major policy issues. Two major issues were discussed: (1) Medicaid does not pay for social work services and many low-income patients really need these services; and (2) social work is not a skilled, independent service as nursing and physical therapy are; thus, the social worker cannot stay on a case where the nurse and therapist have discharged the patient. This causes premature discharge, rehospitalization, and/ or inadequate discharge planning.

Implications for Future Applications

Social Work Practice

This study and its findings have serious implications for home health social workers in several areas. Social workers who are providing care to patients and their families must possess good skills in performing various tasks, such as psychosocial assessment, counseling and decision making, discharge planning, community resources, and supervision. They also must have the ability to be flexible, independent, personable, and able to enter unpredictable—sometimes marginal—situations. Also, the study points to a serious need for social workers to be team players and to be an active part of an interdisciplinary health care team. This is especially true in home health care, because nursing and physical therapy are primary service providers. Social work is a secondary role, and social workers must be visible, assertive, and active within agencies.

Home Health Care Providers

The investigator feels that this study will have tremendous impact on home health care providers. The study points to a serious lack of knowledge among agencies about social work services. Home health care administrators must take a more active role in learning about social work and in developing resources. Agencies need to develop more educational programs in the home health and social work areas, such as conducting workshops and seminars, along with forming alliances with schools of social work. Because most states have licensure and continuing education requirements, social workers are very receptive to working with agencies on educational pursuits. It is suggested that each state's council on home health care sponsor social work-related programs in order to educate providers. In addition, the study demonstrates a tremendous need for social workers with an expertise in home health care, to make themselves available to provide consultation and education services to providers. Home health care agencies currently utilize many consultants.

Social Work Education

The study points to crucial issues for professional social work education and schools of social work. There is a real need for social work programs to incorporate a home health care component into their health care curriculum. Currently, very little attention is being given to home health care, and this could be contributing to the fact that social workers are not being attracted to the field. Also, students are not encouraged to do their undergraduate or graduate field placement training in home health care agencies. Both graduate and undergraduate programs need to develop liaisons with home health care providers to train students and develop continuing education programs.

U.S. News and World Report (Friedman, Hawkins, and Wright, 1994) published a career guide that lists home health care as a "hot track" for social workers. The article points to a serious need for more home health care social workers. To meet this need, there must be more trained social workers.

Policy Issues

The study has several major policy implications. The first issue is that Medicaid still does not reimburse for social work services. This prevents low-income, needy patients from having access to services. Home health care is a medical, cost-driven system. Therefore, agencies only provide services for which they are being reimbursed. The second major issue is whether social work needs to be converted to a skilled independent service, resulting in the social worker being able to enter and leave a case when he or she deems it necessary.

The third major issue is the lack of providers' knowledge about the policies and rules regarding social work services, visits, reimbursement, and staffing regulations. The National Association of Social Workers needs to draw more attention to home health care and develop a national task force. The fourth major issue is that a comprehensive, long-term health care strategy still needs to be developed. Many long-term care services are still not available for a large number of patients.

Implications for Future Research

This study turned out to be a stimulating and worthwhile exploratory endeavor and presented the author an opportunity to address a crucial area of social work. Home health care will continue to expand, and there is a need for more research and scholarly publications in this area.

As for future research possibilities, it is important to look at two other areas: patients' perceptions and beliefs about social workers, and how social workers perceive themselves working in home health care. Social workers, looking beyond the year 2000, must be prepared personally and professionally to practice in this expanding area. They must be able to meet the demands of home health care, respective of their professional goals, ethics, patient and societal values, and personal integrity.

Chapter 3

Problem Areas for Clinical Intervention

During my home care travels, I have worked with clients who exhibited many socioeconomic and psychological problems. Often, the presenting problems for referrals were symptoms of further problems. In reviewing problem areas of hundreds of clients, sixteen major problem areas emerge that require clinical social work intervention and use of community services. I discuss each of these areas from three angles: (1) assessment, (2) intervention, and (3) suggested community service referrals to consider:

- Adjustment to illness
- Terminal illness
- Dementia and behavior management
- Caregiver issues
- Suspected abuse or neglect
- Family conflict
- Placement/alternate housing
- Financial concerns
- Discharge planning
- Inadequate living arrangements/safety and level of care issues
- Substance abuse/chemical dependency
- Social isolation
- Mental health issues
- Legal issues
- Noncompliance with treatment
- Crisis management

tors can be clues that self-neglect or abuse
e environment. Neglect and abuse, either
regiver, are often silent epidemics. When a
al sees these warning signs, a referral to
ces is mandated, by law, in most states.

ORK VISITS AND STAFFING

Visits and Duration
nent

has no minimum or maximum number of
s long as the documentation justifies it.
diaries are looking closely at overutiliza-
vices. They are currently reimbursing only

quires either a master's level social worker
SWE college or university, or a bachelor's
from an accredited college or university,
an MSW.

PROBLEM AREAS

nctioning (e.g., amputation, loss of sight,
loss of speech, new diagnosis, or adjust-

.

Intervention

- Assess and identify transition issues that impact client's management of illness
- Educate client on need for appropriate techniques and resources to comply with plan of care
- Educate client on factors that create emotional, physical, and social changes
- Provide short-term counseling and support

Goals

- Improve client's recovery and plan of care
- Improve client's attitude, self-esteem, and adjustment to new changes and lifestyle

Suggested Referrals/Community Resources

- Support groups
- Mental health agencies
- Day treatment program
- Telephone reassurance
- Disease-specific organizations

Terminal Illness

Problem

Grief, loss, impending death, death, and concerns about dying.

Intervention

- Assess client and family/caregiver's knowledge of end-of-life issues, and ability to cope
- Assess client's condition, support system, and ability to deal with issues

- Educate and provide information and necessary referrals for services such as advance directives, wills, power of attorney, funeral plans, and financial planning
- Provide counseling, emotional support, and improve understanding of grief and loss issues

Goals

- Improve client's self-esteem and confidence
- Improve ability to cope
- Improve family's ability to cope with grief and loss
- Increase client and family knowledge of community resources and services

Suggested Referrals/Community Resources

- Support groups
- Churches
- Hospice programs
- Advance directive forms
- Funeral services
- Financial services

Dementia and Behavior Management

Problem

Dementia and/or behavior that affects medical treatment, quality of life, and safety.

Intervention

- Assess client and caregiver's ability to follow plan of care
- Assess safety, emotional status, and support system
- Assess type of dementia or behavior and its origin, etiology, and needed treatments

- Assess most appropriate long-term care plan
- Assess appropriate goals

Goals

- Provide education and long-term planning on options, environment, placement, or services
- Increase family/caregiver's ability to cope with client's behavior
- Improve quality of life

Suggested Referrals/Community Resources

- Alzheimer's association
- Wandering alert devices
- Personal emergency response system
- Casework agencies
- Support groups
- Respite
- Placement
- Medicaid waiver program

Caregiver Issues

Problem

Caregiver stress, caregiver burdens, and crises such as relocation, hospitalization, illness, and death.

Intervention

- Assess behavior, functioning, mental status, motivation, compliance, and physical health of caregiver
- Assess ability to care for client
- Assess overall management of client
- Assess for needed services

- Provide education on services available to strengthen caregiver's ability to care for clients
- Provide counseling, emotional support, and decision making regarding options

Goals

- Resolve or improve caregiver problems that affect client's condition or recovery
- Reduce caregiver stress and strengthen family care unit
- Reduce management problems and improve client's care

Suggested Referrals/Community Resources

- Support groups
- Respite care
- Mental health services
- Churches
- Medicaid waiver program

Suspected Abuse/Neglect

Problem

Alleged or suspected abuse and/or neglect.

Intervention

- Assess risks and mental/physical status of client and caregiver (if applicable)
- Assess client's affect, mood, compliance, safety, and family dynamics
- Assess caregiver stress, social and emotional factors, and coping ability
- Evaluate safety and sanitation: smoke alarms, plumbing, water, utilities, clutter, insect infestation, and housing

- Provide education on services to improve client and family functioning
- Provide decision making and long-term planning to facilitate best long-term plan
- Assess mental status/competency of client
- Educate client and family about mental health services available

Goals

- Decrease stressors that will enhance family/client recovery
- Improve safety and decrease risks
- Improve coping
- Appropriate long-term plan
- Appropriate living arrangement

Suggested Referrals/Community Resources

- Support groups
- Homemaker services
- Adult protective services (mandated referral)
- Respite services
- Mental health programs
- Meals-on-wheels
- Medicaid waiver program

High-Risk Screening Factors for Possible Abuse and Neglect

- Unexplained bruises or burns
- Inadequate nutrition
- Deteriorated housing
- Insect-infested housing
- Financial exploitation
- Clients left alone who are severely impaired
- Clients lying in urine or feces

- Severely mentally and physically impaired and living alone
- Isolation and reclusiveness
- Sensory deprivation
- Substandard housing: inadequate heat, poor ventilation, inadequate insulation, improper plumbing
- Caregiver depending on parent's income
- Poor family dynamics: yelling, screaming, hitting
- Leaving medical care against medical advice (AMA)
- Individuals who appear passive, fearful, anxious
- Clients unable to make appropriate decisions
- Failure to thrive
- Caregiver stress and burden
- Alcohol and/or drug abuse
- Continuous abnormal blood sugar levels, temperature, urinary tract infections, etc.
- Unexplained fractures, falls

Figure 3.1 is a worksheet that can be used as a tool to document abuse and neglect incidents for Adult Protective Services.

Family Conflict

Problem

Family conflict that negatively affects the client's condition or plan of treatment.

Intervention

- Assess client's short-term goals, family dynamics, and family factors causing the conflict
- Provide short-term counseling and long-term planning
- Educate client and family on community services to provide a solution and resolution of the conflict

(Note: Medicare only allows two to three visits for this activity.)

FIGURE 3.1. Documentation Worksheet

File number: _____

Patient's name: _____

Employee reporting incident classification: _____

Description of incident: _____

_____

_____

_____

Date reported to Adult Protective Services: _____

Name of person taking referral: _____

Follow-up: _____

_____

_____

_____

_____

_____

Goal

- Increase client and family understanding of the dynamics of their conflict and resources to decrease it

Suggested Referrals/Community Resources

- Family counseling
- Casework agencies
- Golden age centers
- Mental health centers
- Adult protective services
- Respite programs
- Day care

Placement/Alternate Housing

Problem

Client is in need of alternate placement, that is, long-term care, assisted living, or protective setting.

Intervention

- Complete initial psychosocial assessment
- Assess client's ability to remain in his or her own home
- Assess medical factors, mental status, support system, and financial resources
- Assess social support system and caregiver's ability to handle client's needs
- Assess need for possible urgent placement
- Assess level of care, services needed, and financial resources
- Hold a family conference, if possible, to discuss options, decision making, and financial arrangements

- Educate client and family and provide written listings and directions of long-term care/housing options and fees
- Arrange for level of care determination, if required in your state, and instruct family on financial arrangements and advanced directions if needed

Goals

- To make sure client has an appropriate long-term care plan
- An appropriate placement or housing plan for client's needs to be met

Suggested Referrals/Community Resources

- Nursing home facilities
- Assisted living facilities
- Day care facilities
- Respite care
- Group homes
- Family care homes
- Senior apartments
- Emergency personal alarm system

Financial Concerns

Problem

Financial issues that create stress, anxiety, and negatively affect the client's ability to comply with treatment plan

Intervention

- Assess client's treatment plan and financial stressors affecting it
- Assess client's income versus expenses, credit obligations, medical bills, and housing/utilities

- Assess client's ability to purchase medications, prescriptions, supplies, and equipment
- Assess client's eligibility for Medicare and Medicaid
- Complete needed documents to enroll client in necessary pharmaceutical programs
- Educate client on community resources

(Note: HCFA does not pay for social work home visits to complete Medicaid application. The social worker can assist clients applying for benefits.)

Goals

- To reduce or relieve financial stress
- To assist client in obtaining necessary medications, supplies, and equipment
- To enhance client's compliance with treatment plan

Suggested Referrals/Community Resources

- Subsidized housing
- Pharmaceutical programs
- Emergency assistance programs
- Medicaid
- Medication samples from physicians' offices
- Disease-specific associations
- American Cancer Society
- Durable Medical Equipment (DME) companion
- Social Security Administration

Discharge Planning

Problem

Make appropriate transition from home health care agency and ensure client's needs are met through linkage to other community services. (Note: It is expected that with the emergence of prospective payment, discharge planning will be a major activity area.)

Intervention

- Assess client's level of functioning, ADL status, and needs upon discharge
- Assess client's understanding of his/her needs, financial resources, and ability to access services
- Assist client, caregivers, and family in developing an in-home care system and safety plan
- Educate and instruct client and family on community resources and services available and how to access them
- Provide and refer to appropriate service linkages

(Note: provide written instruction, name, and phone number of contact person, agencies, and service plan.)

Goals

- Appropriate long-term care plan with necessary linkages to needed services
- To ensure client's safety after agency discharge; improve client/caregiver knowledge of community resources

Suggested Referrals/Community Resources

- Income assistance programs
- Continued personal care programs
- Transportation services
- Nutrition and meals programs
- Home repair programs
- Housekeeping/chore services
- Mental health services

- Casework agencies
- Support groups
- Housing options
- Day care
- Medicaid waiver program

Inadequate Living Arrangements/Safety and Level of Care Issues

Problem

Physical, emotional, social, or home environment issues that negatively affect client's safety; need for increased care/supervision.

Intervention

- Assess client's current and past ADL functioning
- Assess client's safety and ability to remain in home
- Assess the possible need for alternative placement
- Assess care needs, stressors, and ability to manage at home
- Assess legal and financial needs
- Educate and instruct client and family on needed community services or placement options, if indicated
- Refer client to services to enhance safety and reduce risk factors

Goals

- Define and reduce safety risks
- Provide and ensure an appropriate long-term plan for protection and safety
- Appropriate linkage to needed services

Suggested Referrals/Community Resources

- Medicaid waiver program
- Police departments

- Fire departments
- Medic alert program
- DME supplies and home equipment
- Respite
- In-home care services
- Alternate placement options

Substance Abuse/Chemical Dependency

Problem

The abuse of alcohol or drugs, which negatively affects client's mental or physical health or plan of care.

Intervention

- Assess whether client or caregiver is currently in danger
- Coordinate appropriate intervention, if danger exists
- Educate client/family on substance abuse and its effects
- Link to appropriate community resources

(Note: This area of activity must be short term and is usually done in conjunction with other activities, such as discharge planning.)

Goal

- To ensure client's safety and/or improve his or her functioning and rate of recovery

Suggested Referrals/Community Resources

- Self-help groups
- Alcohol and drug agencies or programs
- Inpatient or outpatient substance abuse treatment
- Adult protective services (if needed)

Social Isolation

Problem

Lack of social supports, lack of social stimulation, reclusiveness.

Intervention

- Assess current support system
- Educate and instruct client on community services to decrease isolation
- Assess client's mental status, physical status, and ability to remain in current living environment
- Make alternative living arrangements, if necessary

Goals

- To establish a network of social supports and community services to reduce isolation in current environment
- Obtain alternate placement

Suggested Referrals/Community Resources

- Private duty sitter or companion
- Transportation services
- Telephone reassurance programs
- Friendly visits
- Personal emergency response system
- Casework agencies
- Medicaid waiver program

Mental Health Issues

Problem

Emotional and psychological aspects of illness that will negatively affect treatment plan. (Note: This activity area requires the skills of an MSW and in some states, licensure as an independent, or advanced clinical status.)

Intervention

- Complete a psychosocial assessment
- Assess for previous psychiatric history
- Assess mental status
- Assess response to illness
- Assess current coping ability
- Assess any current psychiatric problems
- Assess clinical symptoms and findings for depression; anxiety disorder, such as panic, phobia, obsessive-compulsive disorder; schizophrenia; psychotic disorder; dementia; substance abuse; suicidal ideation
- Provide short-term therapy for loss of independence with reduced ADL functioning, ineffective coping skills, altered body image, conflict resolution, adjustment to illness

Goals

- Improve ability to cope with illness and reduced functioning
- Provide appropriate mental health linkage for long-term follow-up

Suggested Referral/Community Resources

- Psychiatric home care programs
- Community mental health centers
- Counseling agencies
- Disease-specific services

Legal Issues

Problem

The need for education and resource linkage to legal services. (Note: This activity must be completed in conjunction with discharge planning.)

Intervention

- Provide education and linkage to the following:
  — living will
  — durable health care power of attorney
  — financial power of attorney
  — representative payer
  — Adult Protective Services
  — guardianship
- Provide documents—but it is highly advisable not to sign or witness them
- Refer client and/or family to appropriate legal consultation, such as Elder Law, Health Care law

Suggested Referrals/Community Resources

- Legal Aid
- Elder Law attorneys
- Health Care attorneys
- AARP Legal Hotline
- Office of Aging

Noncompliance with Treatment

Problem

Client does not follow health care treatment plan.

Intervention

- Assess factors contributing to noncompliance:
  — Financial resources
  — History
  — Personality
  — Family conflict
  — Support system
- Provide education and linkage for follow-up

Goal

- Increase compliance and achieve medically desired results

Referrals

- Financial resources
- Counseling
- Mental health agencies

CRISIS MANAGEMENT

All crises, accidents, or incidents that occur in the field are to be reported to the director of nursing or clinical services immediately by phone. These include accidents, falls, medical emergencies, altercations, complaints, suicidal ideation, homicidal ideation, and abuse. All crises and incidents must be put in writing and documented thoroughly.

For suicidal ideation, client must be assessed immediately and should be referred to a psychiatric emergency unit, a mental health crisis team, or a hospital emergency room. Also, a referral to the suicide hotline and police is indicated. Use Suicide Lethality Scale to assess harm potential and mental status and document results.

For homicidal ideation, the police should be notified, plus Adult Protective Services if the client is elderly. In all mental health emergencies, provide short-term crisis counseling and linkage to mental health resources. Document everything you observe, your assessment, and your actions. Do not leave client's environment until crisis is resolved and he or she is in another treatment setting.

Suicide Behavior Screening and Assessment Factors

1. Inquire about presence of suicidal ideation

   • Note frequency, intensity, duration
   • Ego-alien (seems foreign) or ego-syntonic (consistent with self)
   • Presence of command hallucinations requires an immediate psychiatric consultation

2. Inquire about presence and nature of plan

   • Are means of implementing plan readily available?
   • Determine how easy it would be to follow through with plan

3. Is individual showing signs of impulsivity?
4. Does the individual have a weapon or ready access to one?
5. Key predictor: history of prior attempts

   • How many?
   • Nature of attempts: high lethality (jumping off bridge) versus low lethality (gestures such as scraping wrist with potato peeler)
   • Was failure of previous attempts unlikely or serendipitous?
   • Pattern with multiple attempts (e.g., increase in lethality)

6. Assess degree of depression

   • Vegetative disturbance
   • Feelings of hopelessness/futility
   • Agitation or its resolution into a sense of calm

7. Assess recent losses: significant others, roles, etc.
8. Has individual given up key possessions or "made peace"?
9. Is individual willing to sign a no-suicide contract?
10. Will individual agree to follow-up care/reschedule?
11. Note that individuals who intend to merely gesture for help sometimes make mistakes and die
12. Listen to your gut instincts
13. Do not hesitate to consult with another or ask for help
14. Assess the adequacy of the individual's support system
15. With adolescents, watch for copycat suicides, either with celebrity suicides, or especially with teen suicides in a geographic area
16. Substance use and withdrawal are risk factors, especially with crack and alcohol

Chapter 4

Staffing Models

Home health agencies may or may not choose to offer social work services.

At the time this book was written, home health agencies were moving toward employing master's degree social workers because of their ability to function independently and utilize skills in complex cases. Also, many home health clients have multiple medical and psychiatric problems. Certified psychiatric home care programs must employ master's degree and licensed independent social workers because only they are permitted to assess and treat mental disorders. Some agencies successfully employ BSW social workers with supervision provided by an MSW social worker.

The following job descriptions serve as a guide to agencies for MSW- and BSW-level social workers.

JOB DESCRIPTIONS FOR MSW- AND BSW-LEVEL SOCIAL WORKERS

Medical Social Worker—Master's Degree

Job Summary

The medical social worker prepares social histories; provides social casework to patients and families having difficulty in social functioning; aids in the referral process; and generally serves as a social worker in the agency's total program in order to supplement overall patient care.

Qualifications

1. Master's degree in social work required
2. Licensed, registered, or certified by the State Board of Social Work Examiners of the state in which the medical social worker resides or practices (if applicable)
3. Preferably two years' experience in medical social work, home health, homemaker services, or services to the aged or ill
4. Experience and ability in family assessment
5. Ability to work with other health care professionals in the home health industry

Position Responsibilities

1. Provides social casework, when appropriate, to individuals and families receiving nursing or other services from the agency
2. Prepares social histories according to specific guidelines to augment existing service, or as a guide in determining or changing level of service, taking into consideration:

   • Family relationships
   • The meaning of illness to the patient and family
   • The cultural attitudes in relation to illness
   • The meaning of home to the patient
   • The ability of the patient and his or her family to adjust to the patient at home
   • The financial impact of illness upon the family

3. Assesses, when appropriate, a family's financial situation, taking into consideration the patient's prognosis and medical needs, and referring the family to an agency for financial assistance if necessary, interpreting the medical situation to the referring agency and generally facilitating the process of referral
4. Responds to referrals for casework by agency staff or professionals from outside the agency providing service as appropriate

5. Participates in agency team conferences identifying social problems, their severity, and their interrelatedness to the medical situation, as well as assessing a family's strengths and weaknesses and discussing alternate methods of alleviating the situation
6. Refers patients and families to community agencies with appropriate follow-up
7. Participates in case conferences with other agencies
8. Interprets social resources to staff and health services to special agencies
9. Maintains absolute confidentiality of agency records, including, but not limited to, payroll, personnel, patient care, business plans, and financial information
10. Maintains absolute confidentiality of patient's records
11. Assists the physician and other team members in understanding significant social and emotional factors related to patient's health problems
12. Participates in the development of a treatment plan
13. Observes the patient, and records and reports information on the patient's condition to the attending physician and in the patient's health record
14. Advises, counsels, and, when appropriate, instructs the family in the patient's social needs
15. Participates in discharge planning
16. Participates in in-service education programs
17. Supervises bachelor-degree social workers and co-signs their patient notes; adheres to all rules, regulations, codes of ethics, guidelines, and codes in federal, state, and local laws that are concerned with the practice of medical social work; adheres to the policies established by the agency
18. Performs other job-related duties as assigned

Relationships

The medical social worker reports to the agency administrator or director.

Medical Social Worker—Bachelor's Degree

Job Summary

The medical social worker is a qualified professional who provides medical social services to patients in their homes with physician's orders and under the direction of a master's degree social worker.

Qualifications

1. Bachelor's degree graduate of a school of social work approved by the Council on Social Work Education preferred
2. Minimum one year prior experience in a medical setting (hospital, clinic, rehabilitation center, etc.) where the team approach to treatment was utilized
3. Currently licensed by state board of social workers
4. Ability to travel extensively, during all seasons, to clients' homes and to work in various home environments
5. Working knowledge of community resources and various social service systems

Responsibilities

1. Clinical responsibilities
   - Provides rehabilitative and supportive casework geared to restoring patients to their optimum level of social and health adjustments. This includes assisting patients and their families in understanding, accepting, and following medical recommendations.
   - Helps patients utilize the resources of their families and communities. This may be accomplished by either referring patients to resources or acting as an intermediary on behalf of the patients in their dealings with other health and welfare agencies.

- Assists patients and their families with personal and environmental difficulties that predispose them toward illness or interfere with obtaining maximum benefits from medical care. This may range from counseling family members to assisting the patient with admission to a nursing home.
- Consults with physicians and other members of the health team for the purpose of helping them to understand significant social, emotional, and environmental factors related to the patient's health problems.
- Participates in client case conferences and service team meetings, as required.
- Participates in staff development activities and acts as consultant to other agency personnel.
- Participates in the development of a treatment plan, care plan, and discharge planning.
- Submits clinical and progress notes in accordance with agency policies and procedures.

2. General responsibilities
- Promotes harmonious relationships and favorable attitudes between clients and staff.
- Supports and adheres to organizational policies, procedures, philosophies, and goals at all times.
- Maintains confidentiality of agency, staff, and client information.
- Assists clients, personnel, and visitors, as needed.
- Represents the agency in a loyal and professional manner, at all times.
- Performs other duties as assigned.

It is crucial that the social worker and the home health agency review their state's licensing and credentialing standards for social workers before deciding on social work personnel standards. Also, often master's degree social workers are still licensed at the bachelor level. This could present a potential problem, especially in providing social work services to mental health-related clients.

Chapter 5

Clinical Patient Care Policies Regarding Social Work Services

INTRODUCTION

Licensed social workers assist individuals and their families to identify, resolve, or minimize problems that often accompany illness.

Personnel Involved

Social services are provided by a person with a master's degree in social work accredited by the Council on Social Work Education. Services may also be performed by a licensed social worker with a bachelor's degree in social work, under the supervision of the master's level social worker.

Scope of Service

Social work services are provided in the home setting to persons who have met the eligibility requirements and have been accepted for care by the agency.

Limitations

A treatment plan must be established by the physician to authorize medical social services. Nursing or physical therapy services must be active with a patient and identify needs that require medical social service intervention. When these needs have been identified, a request for social work evaluation can be made to the supervisor of the agency. The referring discipline and social service then coordinate their services by conferring about the identified needs. Therefore, social service intervention is anticipated to be of short duration and provides the link to minimize social problems and determine methods of implementing community resources.

NATURE OF SERVICES

Medical social services assist in providing continuity of patient care in the following ways:

1. Providing social case work to help patients with social, emotional, personal, environmental, and financial difficulties that predispose them toward illness or interfere with obtaining maximum benefits from medical care
2. Counseling patients and members of the family about areas of social work intervention to resolve or minimize social pressures, and assist in implementation of these interventions
3. Providing support and counseling to the patient and members of the family in crisis situations, including death
4. Coordinating methods of social work intervention and potential problem areas with all disciplines providing patient care
5. Providing emotional support to the patient and members of the family to help them handle their feelings, gain acceptance of the illness or disability, and to assist them in using their personal strengths toward recovery goals, which often includes adjusting interpersonal roles and modification of lifestyles
6. Collaborating with community agencies and making appropriate referrals for additional services

RESPONSIBILITIES

1. Assisting the physician and other team members in understanding significant social and emotional factors related to health problems

2. Participate in the development of a plan of treatment and necessary progress reports
3. Prepare clinical notes
4. Coordinate social services plans and goals with other disciplines active in the care of the client
5. Utilize appropriate community resources
6. Work directly and indirectly with the family
7. Participate in discharge planning and in-service programs
8. Act as a consultant to other personnel

PROCEDURE FOR IMPLEMENTATION OF MEDICAL SOCIAL SERVICES

Basic areas of need should be identified prior to social service involvement and these needs may relate to:

• Information, education, and supportive services
• Counseling concerning adjustment to illness/disability
• Referrals to medical and nonmedical community agencies
• Arranging outpatient medical and nonmedical support
• Transportation
• Financial counseling
• Protective and/or inpatient legal services
• Protective living arrangements
• Institutional placement

All requests for medical social work must be authorized by the primary physician prior to the evaluation visit.

This authorization may be included in the original request for home care services. However, any professional member of the home care team may identify the need for social services if they were not originally ordered by the physician. The team member is responsible for contacting the primary physician to obtain verbal approval, followed by written authorization, and notifying the administrator of the secured authorization.

Visitation Schedule

The supervisor assigns the case to a licensed social worker, who is accountable and responsible for the evaluation and follow-up visits.

Coordination of Services

The social worker is made aware of the request for service by written referral and is also notified of other team members providing services. The social worker is responsible for contacting workers in other disciplines to collaborate on identified needs, implementation plans, and goals.

The supervisor is verbally made aware of any case difficulties. The patient's ongoing progress is noted by a review of documentation submitted for the medical record. The master's degree social worker has a conference with the bachelor's degree social worker and co-signs all visit notes, physician orders, and conference notes.

Documentation

The social worker is accountable for completing documentation on the date of the home visit and submitting documentation for inclusion in the clinical record on a weekly basis. Documentation responsibilities include:

- Evaluation/assessment
- Development of the plan of treatment
- Problems/needs
- Goals (short-term and long-term)
- Care plan formulation and implementation
- Clinical note and progress report (medical update)
- Conference records
- Discharge summary, including services offered, patient/ family responses, and disposition of case

Documentation must consist of problem-oriented recording in terms of problems, interventions, and outcomes. There are three major areas for intervention, depending on the individual, social situation, and/or disease process.

Problems	Interventions	Outcomes
Increased stress from illness due to decreased physical/mental functioning, role changes, family conflict, change in body image, dependency needs, demanding behavior.	• Give adequate information. • Explore behavioral/ thinking patterns with patient/family to help patient/family accept disease process and physical/mental changes. • Mediate family conflict. • Encourage independence and/or acceptance of dependency needs. • Help family set limits.	Increased ability to cope with stress, and thereby improve patient and family's ability to comply with care plan in order to help patient recover and regain independence.
Financial difficulties due to illness resulting in increased anxiety and failure to obtain medicine, food, heat, medical treatment, or transportation.	• Budget overview and planning. • Explain insurance, and teach patient and family to fill out insurance forms. • Utilize outside resources for financial assistance.	Decreased anxiety. Obtain appropriate medical care, drugs and food. Patient is able to recover and regain independence.
Unsafe or inadequate living arrangements for patient.	• Give information to patient and family to fill out insurance forms. • Utilize outside resources for financial assistance. • Refer to community services.	Clear decision on what is best for patient/family and to restore an environment conducive to achieving maximum independence and health.

SOCIAL WORK ROLES AND RESPONSIBILITIES

There are four major areas of social work services in home health care agencies:

- Assessment of social and emotional factors
- Counseling for decision making and long-term planning
- Community resources planning
- Short-term therapy

Other areas include environmental/living situation and risks and safety factors, assistance with financial problems, alternative placement planning, and crisis intervention. Each of these areas will now be discussed in more detail.

Assessment of Social and Emotional Factors

- Response to diagnosis and illness
- Need for care
- Loss of independence
- Response to treatment
- Support systems

Goal

The goal is to improve patient/caregiver knowledge of social/ emotional factors adversely affecting response to illness.

Counseling for Long-Range Planning/Decision Making

- Evaluate home situation
- Assist in alternate living arrangements
- Assist in extended care facility (ECF) placement
- Assist in ensuring safe environment
- Improve coping with disease limitations to accept needed assistance

Goal

The goal is to improve patient/caregiver knowledge of long-term planning and decision making regarding alternate living arrangements, ECF placement, and needs for additional in-home assistance.

Community Resource Planning

- Income assistance program
- Housekeeping/chore services
- Continued personal care assistance
- Obtaining adequate transportation
- Support groups regarding adjustment to disease
- Obtaining adequate food
- Obtaining adequate medication
- Obtaining assistance with needed home repair
- Placement in long-term therapy

Goal

The goal is to improve patient/caregiver knowledge of appropriate community resources and to help in their effective utilization.

Short-Term Therapy with Goal-Oriented Intervention

- Loss of independence with decreased ADL status
- Management of terminal illness
- Ineffective coping skills, adjustment to illness
- Altered body image
- Nonacceptance of diagnosis interfering with accepting needed assistance from family/support system
- Conflict resolution related to chronic illness

Goal

The goal is to improve ability to cope regarding management of illness, diagnosis and prognosis, loss of independence with decreased ADL status, acceptance of necessary role reversal with family support systems, and altered body image.

Environment/Living Situation Assessment

Current patient living arrangements:

- Own home
- Apartment
- Senior citizen apartment
- Significant other's home

Patient lives:

- Alone
- With spouse
- With adult child

ADL needs currently met by:

- Patient
- Patient with assistance from caregiver
- Caregiver providing complete care
- Care is adequate or inadequate

Meal preparation needs met by:

- Patient
- Patient with assistance from caregiver
- Caregiver providing complete meal preparation
- Meal preparation is adequate or inadequate

Housekeeping/chore services provided by:

- Patient with assistance from others
- Others providing chore services
- Not being provided

Home environment:

- Clean
- Sanitation problems
- Lack of heat
- Lack of water
- Insect infested
- Inadequate chore provider
- Lack of basic home appliances
- Home environment safe or unsafe

Assistance with Financial Problems

- Needs referral to prescription program for indigent persons
- Referral to food stamp program
- Referral to Medicaid assistance
- Referral to Social Security disability program
- Referral to financial entitlement program
- Referral to crisis food bank or hunger center
- Intervention with electric and/or gas company to prevent shutoff

Alternative Placement Planning

Client needs placement in:

- Group home
- Assisted living
- Foster home
- ICF nursing home
- ECF nursing home
- Hospice center
- Respite center
- Senior housing
- Relocation due to substandard housing

Clinical Findings for Crisis Intervention

Signs and Symptoms of Serious Depression:

- Withdrawn, isolation
- Appetite disturbance
- Sleep problems
- Suicidal ideation
- Homicidal ideation
- Child abuse
- Others, i.e., severe dementia, schizophrenia, or paranoia

May need to refer client to a twenty-four-hour mobile crisis team.

Chapter 6

Appropriate Clients
for Social Work Intervention

In a home health care agency, social work is not an independent skilled service and only the RN, case manager, or physical therapist can obtain a physician's order and refer a client. Since social work service is not primary and most health care professionals are not trained in agencies to screen clients, social work remains a drastically underutilized area of service. Nurses, in particular, need to be trained on how to screen their clients for factors or characteristics that need social work intervention. The utilization of social work service is directly related to how well the home health care staff are trained to understand the social work role and how social work service can benefit their clients.

In 1991, to assist in screening clients, an NASW Home Care Task Force developed the following list of client factors that indicate a need for social work intervention (NASW, 1991):

- Patients in need of a skilled assessment of social and emotional factors affecting their illnesses or treatment plans
- Patients who have suffered a sudden loss of physical functions with an impact on treatment management, e.g., cerebral vascular accident (CVA), amputation, heart attack, Parkinson's disease, multiple sclerosis, or acute loss of sight, hearing, or speech
- Patients with terminal illnesses who are experiencing (a) severe loss or anger, and/or (b) family strain and economic difficulties, which weaken their support system

- Patients whose cognitive or behavior problems create difficulty for home management, e.g., Alzheimer's, organic brain syndrome (OBS), organic psychosis
- Patients with high-tech needs whose families are having difficulty managing their care
- Patients who have recently experienced a change in caregiver status (e.g., death or sudden hospitalization of a family member), which interferes with the treatment plan
- Patients who need community resources or information to manage short- and long-term care at home, e.g., housekeeping/chores, financial aid, adult day care, transportation, medical appliances and services, alternative housing, vocational training, friendly visitors, emergency response system, long-term counseling, entitlement programs, assistance with insurance claims, and/or energy assistance
- Patients in need of nursing home or institutional placement
- Patients who are experiencing marital conflicts, which create social problems for themselves and their spouses and impede effective treatment
- Patients at high risk due to any combination of the following: social isolation, decreased mental capacity, lack of informal or formal support systems, unsafe or unstable home environment, suspected neglect or abuse, lack of financial resources, and substance abuse
- Patients in need of advocacy to secure their right to services and benefits
- Patients unwilling or unable to follow treatment plans
- Patients with suicidal ideation
- Patients in need of guardianship or conservatorship

Because of my own home health care travels, I have added several other "red flags" as high-risk screening factors for more serious problems, such as suspected neglect or abuse. For a list of these factors, see Chapter 3.

Chapter 7

Medicare Standards for Social Work Practice in Home Health Care

Medicare is the largest single payer of home health care services. Formal caregivers include professionals and paraprofessionals who provide in-home care, including nursing and personal care.

Unfortunately, the home health care industry is still focused on an illness-driven or medically driven model. According to the National Association of Home Care (1999), over 500,000 individuals are employed in the home health care field, but these employees only convert to about 372,000 full-time equivalent employees. This means that numerous employees are working on an as-needed or PRN basis, part time, or contract only. Most of these full-time employees are registered nurses, representing over 132,000 full-time employees. Another 124,000 are full-time home health aides (National Association of Home Care, 1999).

Social workers represent only a small segment of home health care services. There are approximately 9,000 total social workers in the home care industry, but only about 6,900 represent full-time equivalent employees. This is also now on the decline because visits are decreasing due to the 1997 Balanced Budget Act. Rather than focusing on preventive or holistic care that would lead to more access to services and independence, home care agencies are choosing to focus their costs and spending on nursing and personal care services.

The new Medicare beneficiary cap for each home health client is approximately $3,500 a year, and most of this is being spent on nursing and home health aide service. The funds for home health are not being spent on rehabilitation and social work services, which would assist clients to become more independent.

Social work services are not being utilized along with rehabilitation services because these services are more costly to provide and personnel require a higher per-visit rate. Social work services would greatly benefit patients in that other non-Medicare services could be made more available and discharge planning could be started sooner. Agencies could actually have lower costs, better utilization of services, and faster turnover of new patients as a prospective pay system emerges.

Social work services, therefore, still receive very little attention, and social workers are secondary. The majority of home health care recipients are never referred for social work services and are missing out on numerous services. These crucial services include meals-on-wheels, mental health services, case management, transportation, financial services, Medicaid, day care, assistive devices, assistance in paying for prescriptions, companion services, support groups, legal services, protective services, and many more.

Experts predict that by 2025, the world population will top 8.5 billion and the elderly population will exceed 1.1 billion. As a result, all countries will have to develop long-term services to serve the population. All countries will have to focus on non-Medicare, nonmedical, or noninstitutional care and provide social services and community services as alternatives.

Medical social work services can improve the emotional and social well-being of patients and expand their long-term options. Social work reduces overall treatment costs. A multidisciplinary approach is crucial.

MEDICARE STANDARDS
ON SOCIAL WORK SERVICES

- Currently, Medicare requires all social work visits and activities to be directly related to the overall medical treatment of the client.

- Financial counseling and assistance must be related to the medical treatment of the client, i.e., nutrition, prescriptions, supplies, and to improve compliance.
- Visits to complete Medicare applications are not covered. A social worker can refer and assist clients in applying.
- There is no minimum or maximum number of visits that are allowed or reimbursed. Every visit must stand on its own merit. Every visit must be medically justified and documentation must be appropriate.
- Generally, one to four visits will be covered. Exceptions are placements, crisis intervention, abuse or neglect, and relocation.

MEDICAL SOCIAL SERVICES

Medical social services that are provided by a qualified medical social worker (MSW), or a social work assistant (BSW) under the supervision of a qualified MSW, may be covered as home health services where the patient meets the qualifying criteria (Health Care Financing Administration, 1992):

- The services of these professionals are necessary to resolve social or emotional problems that are expected to be impediments to the effective treatment of the patient's medical condition or his or her rate of recovery.
- The plan of care indicates how the services that are required necessitate the skills of a qualified social worker or a social work assistant under the supervision of a qualified medical social worker to be performed safely and effectively.

If both requirements for coverage are met, professional services covered include, but are not limited to, the following:

- Assessment of the social and emotional factors related to the patient's illness, need for care, response to treatment, and adjustment to care.

- Assessment of the relationship of the patient's medical and nursing requirements to the patient's home situation, financial resources, and availability of community resources.
- Appropriate action to obtain available community resources to assist in resolving the patient's problem. (Note: Medicare does not cover the services of a medical social worker to complete or assist in the completion of an application for Medicaid, because federal regulations require the state to provide assistance in completing the application to anyone who chooses to apply for Medicaid.)
- Counseling services required by the patient.
- Medical social services provided to the patient's family member or caregiver on a short-term basis when the HHA can demonstrate that a brief intervention (i.e., two or three visits) by a medical social worker is necessary to remove a clear and direct impediment to the effective treatment of the patient's medical condition or to his or her rate of recovery. To be considered "clear and direct," the behavior or actions of the family member or caregiver must plainly obstruct, contravene, or prevent the patient's medical treatment or rate of recovery. Medical social services to address general problems that do not clearly and directly impede treatment or recovery as well as long-term social services furnished to family members, such as ongoing alcohol counseling, are not covered.

Note: Participation in the development of the plan of care, preparing clinical and progress notes, participating in discharge planning and in-service programs, and acting as a consultant to other agency personnel are appropriate administrative costs to the HHA (Health Care Financing Administration, 1992).

SOCIAL WORK REFERRALS
AND DOCUMENTATION

1. The RN/case manager should first obtain a verbal order from a physician for social work services. Then he or she sends the order to the MD for a signature.
2. Preferably, the RN should refer the client for social work services as soon as the client is ready for services by the agency.
3. The RN should place the client on the 485/HCFA certification plan of care form: MSW, evaluate and treat.
4. The social worker then makes his or her first visit for a social work evaluation and writes his or her own orders.
5. Appropriate orders: two to four MSW visits. Period of dates to do psychosocial assessment, community resource planning, and discharge planning.
6. A certification period begins at the agency's start of care date and lasts for nine weeks.
7. In this nine-week period, the social worker can, if justified, do two to four visits.
8. If the social worker does not do exactly four visits, he or she must write an order, sign it along with the RN, and obtain a signature from the MD.

Appropriate Reasons for the Nurse or Case Manager to Refer Client for Social Work Services

When an RN makes a referral to a social worker, the RN must provide the following:

1. A written verbal order from the medical doctor
2. An interdisciplinary referral form explaining why the social worker is being brought into the case
3. A copy of the 485/plan of care.

An RN can refer clients to a social worker for any of the following reasons:

- Socioemotional factors affecting care and rehabilitation
- Emotional distress, depression, or anxiety
- Discharge planning needs
- Financial concerns
- Lack of knowledge regarding community resources
- Social isolation
- Safety concerns (i.e., adequate or appropriate care in home)
- Needs education or assistance with advance directives
- Family or caregiver concerns
- Crisis intervention or placement needed
- Needs assistance in advocating and negotiating social systems
- Needs advocate for community services for patients at risk due to mental and/or physical limitations
- Needs short-term therapy/counseling

Documentation Protocols After Each Visit

- The assessment visit should be done no later than seventy-two hours after orders are written. Some agencies require twenty-four to forty-eight hours.
- After the first visit, the social worker must complete an evaluation/assessment form and a care plan.
- If the first visit is the only one needed, the social worker writes an order saying "Evaluation Only Needed." The order must be signed by the social worker and the RN.
- If the social worker is opening the case, orders should include two to four visits.
- For follow-up visits, the social worker should complete only the revisit form.
- If the social worker fails to make a visit, the reason must be documented on the appropriate form.
- The social worker should make as many client-related phone calls as possible during the visit and document the client's response and interaction.

DISCHARGE PLANNING

With home care moving to DRGs and prospective payment, discharge planning will soon be the primary role in home health care, which is similar to the discharge planning provided by hospitals. When doing counseling and discharge planning, the following areas need to be assessed:

- Follow-up casework
- Mental health follow-up
- Meals-on-wheels, supplements, diet
- Housing assistance, mobility, supplies
- Prescription assistance
- Continued rehabilitation
- Day care
- Options for long-term care (including a written list of agencies)

COORDINATION OF CARE AND DOCUMENTATION

- Medicare mandates that home health care agencies provide interdisciplinary case planning, discharge planning, and coordination of care.
- Weekly case conferences should be held and all disciplines should be represented. All clients should be discussed on a cycle (determined by the agency) with progress, problems, and plans documented and summarized, and every person attending must sign.
- Also, all phone calls between disciplines and community agencies must be documented to prove coordination of care within and outside the agency.
- All phone calls made by the social worker must be documented on a coordination of care form or a similar form. Each agency can develop its own form.

Quality Assurance

- For social work, there should be a chart audit of 20 percent of active clients and 10 percent of discharged clients.
- The chart audit should be done quarterly and reviewed and co-signed by the social worker and another LISW.
- It is not mandatory, but it is good practice to track adult protective service referrals and follow-up.
- The worksheet and log should be kept in a separate, confidential manual. They should not be placed with the medical records.
- Medicare and Joint Commission on Accreditation of Healthcare Organizations (JCAHO) require a quality assurance program.

Guidelines for Medicare Documentation

The social worker should be as objective and specific as possible, and avoid using the following terms:

- *Monitor/supervise.* Denotes a stable patient—use "assess/evaluate."
- *Healing well.* Denotes why visits should not be made; objectively describe wound (size, drainage, color, odor, depth, etc.).
- *Discuss.* Use terms such as teach, educate, instruct, or demonstrate. "Discuss" does not require the skills of a professional; anyone can discuss.
- *Prevent/prevention.* Not covered.
- *Stable/independent.* Negates medical necessity; document response to treatment.
- *Feeling better.* Subjective and provides reason why visits should be discontinued. Focus on patient's problems/needs.
- *Noncompliant/uncooperative.* Document problems with coping or comprehension as source of referral to psychiatric nurse or social worker.

- *Went to the market.* Negates homebound status. Document equipment, manual assistance, and number of people required for patient to leave home. Describe homebound status once a month. Explain why trips were taken and related to lifestyle or medical necessity.
- *Patient not at home.* Use "no answer to locked door," and document on next visit why patient was not at home.
- *Continue care plan.* On the visit report, specifically describe what the next visit plans are based on, e.g., "assess c/p status of CHF patient."
- *Maintenance.* Never use this word because it negates the necessity of visits; document response to the plan of care.
- *Confused.* Describe disorientation to person, place, or time. Describe ability to follow commands, and short- and long-term recall.
- *Chronic condition.* Describe exacerbation of the chronic condition, as chronic condition indicates stable condition.
- *Reinforce/restructure.* Repetitive instruction will not be covered unless learning difficulties are documented. Use words such as demonstrate, teach, instruct, or educate.
- *Observed.* Use assess or evaluate, as anyone can observe. Skilled observation may be used as a component of patient education to document patient/caregiver return demonstration.

Remember: If it isn't documented, it isn't Medicare reimbursable.

As prospective pay enters the home health arena, documentation will become even more crucial. There have already been drastic reductions in home health care visits and more scrutiny of claims. Drastic Medicare overpayments and millions of dollars of inappropriate claims have been made in home health care. In 1996, 1997, and 1998, many health care agencies decided to close their doors, and many more are currently contemplating the same.

Chapter 8

Review
of Medical Social Work Literature

OVERVIEW

Research regarding social work services in health care has expanded greatly since the mid-1980s. New developments in every sector of the field continue to pose challenges for social workers. These new developments include specific diseases, discharge planning, groups, team-oriented practices, health reform, public policy, education, and home health care. Since 1986, the literature that addresses home health care practice has increased. In Ohio, medical social work prevails as the most rapidly growing home health care service. The Ohio Department of Health (1992) reported an increase of 68 percent, or fifty-four agencies that developed social work as a new service component. In 1991 alone social work services increased by 103 percent.

This literature review explores many areas of social work practice in health care, primarily drawn from social work and nursing journals. Because of the scope of material available in this area, this chapter is grouped into twelve clusters:

1. Home health care services for the elderly
2. Social work practice in the bio-ethical area
3. Health care in the future
4. Medical social work and discharge planning
5. Interdisciplinary team practice

6. Policy issues
7. Future directions for home health care
8. Medicare standards for social work practice
9. Health care reform
10. Group work by social workers
11. Disease-specific social work practice
12. Social work practice in home health care

HOME HEALTH CARE SERVICES
FOR THE ELDERLY

The aging of America is a trend that is placing serious strain on our health care system. The elderly are the heaviest users of health care in the population. Their care presents an array of issues, such as cost effectiveness, allocation of resources, methods of insurance, and establishment of priorities for research and service delivery.

Information on access to posthospital care has always been a difficult field of study. In 1987, the General Accounting Office conducted a sample survey of 935 Medicare-certified acute care hospitals on problems in discharge planning, of which 93 percent responded. Of those, 97 percent of hospital discharge planners reported having serious problems in placing Medicare patients in skilled nursing facilities. Another 86 percent also reported problems in placing patients with home health care agencies.

Medicare began to influence medical social work in the 1960s. New areas of practice for the elderly began to emerge, including casework and counseling, financial planning and assistance, consultation with physicians, liaison with the community, education and research, outpatient care, home health, and nursing homes. Medicare reimbursement strategies also began to develop (Watts, 1967).

Wattenberg and McGann (1984) stress the need for community-based and hospital-based social workers to assist older patients in completing insurance forms and applications for programs of entitlement, such as Medicare, Medicaid, food stamps, discounts, and other programs.

Most functionally impaired elderly rely exclusively on family and other informal helpers. Wilcox and Tabu (1991) conducted a study on a sample of 100 elderly clients in a statewide home care program. Most of the clients had fragile helping networks and only 18 percent had helping spouses. Implications for social work practice were discussed, especially the role of case management. Kempen and Suurmeijer (1991) conducted another study on home care utilization among the elderly. A Mokken Scale analysis for polychotomous items was used to measure the level of functional limitations and person-bound variables, along with social support variables. The results showed that the primary users of home care services tend to be women, elderly living alone, and persons living on low incomes. Nonusers receive more informal and private care.

Considerable attention has also been given to the care of demented elderly in the community. Bjorkhem and colleagues (1992) conducted a study on the impact of dementia on caregivers. An interview was conducted with caregivers in questionnaire form. Caregivers expressed a need for training in handling disruptive behaviors, how to stimulate and provide activities for the affected spouse, and for guidance on services available. This is a crucial role for community-based social workers (Levande, Bowden, and Mollema, 1987).

BIOETHICAL ISSUES

Bernstein (1980) outlined legal principles and issues commonly facing social workers, such as the right to a natural death, anatomical gifts, power of attorney, joint bank accounts, wills, insurance, and estates. Social workers play important roles when such legal issues arise, by providing useful information and referrals, as well as by facilitating coping strategies with complex issues at a time of stress for patient and family.

Gelman (1986) considered decisions involving prolongation of life and the participation of the social worker in those decisions. Both Gelman (1986) and Reamer (1985) advocated the establishment of a hospital ethics committee on which social workers could play an active role. Those who understand the dynamics of life-and-death situations can support the patient and family.

HEALTH CARE IN THE FUTURE

Literature on predictions for health care in the future is plentiful. The major conceptual areas are discussed here, and Capra (1982) summarizes some of these predictions.

Numerous diseases—such as high blood pressure, seizures, ulcers, impotence, headaches, arthritis, cardiac arrhythmia, and others—are treated with biofeedback. Various approaches have been attempted, such as yoga, meditation, relaxation techniques, autogenic training, running, and listening to music. The body, via the immune system, seems to have its own way of knowing. The late Ida Rolf was the founder of an approach known as body-work, which alters body energy and affects the entire body-mind loop. A new increase in the use of hypnosis to treat pain, perform surgery, treat phobias, and even promote healing was noted. Thus, a renewed interest in healing phenomena occurred. Behavioral medicine departments and holistic health centers developed prayer networks, acupuncture clinics, homeopathy, herbalism, psychic healing, and guided imagery. The humanistic approach was added to medical schools. Old hierarchical distinctions disappeared. Psychiatrists talked to physicians; nurses, social workers, and physical therapists communicated with one another; and even chiropractors began to be recognized. Labor and delivery units became home oriented. The dying were allowed to die with dignity (with services in their own homes). Interest in older people increased and gerontology became a field of study.

Several changes are already in progress: insurance reform, expansion of health care coverage for women and children, prospective payment system for physician services, and movement toward a national health care system less radical than that in Canada. In 1992, it became illegal for doctors to have any financial interest in companies they utilized. Minimal reimbursement was available for certain procedures, such as hysterectomies, because many were performed that were not required. The same holds true today. Finally, more states have developed Medicaid waiver programs to encourage home health care and reduce nursing home spending.

MEDICAL SOCIAL WORK
AND DISCHARGE PLANNING

In the literature on discharge planning and advocacy, there are three broad categories, each of which reflects the knowledge base of practicing social workers: (1) the role and appropriateness of discharge planning and advocacy as a function of professional social work; (2) skills and knowledge required for the practice of discharge planning and advocacy; and (3) evaluation and demonstration of discharge models and approaches.

Externally induced change in the financial status of the institution stimulates internal reconsideration of the roles, responsibilities, and importance of various departments and professions. This change places increased attention on discharge planning as appropriate to the expertise of the social work professional (Schreiber, 1981). Professional knowledge and proficiencies are required for effective discharge planning. The importance of social work advocacy in health care settings increases with the growing pressure to expedite discharge from acute care settings. The emphasis on shortened and less expensive hospitalization n in the quantity of services provided each

g is inextricably tied to developing re-
ospital care of the patient (Lurie, Pinskey,
andman (1981) identifies five stages in the
ocess: assessment, diagnosis, prescription,
evaluation. The social worker's role is to
the psychosocial elements of patient care,
late to discharge planning.
component of discharge planning is help-
future needs at a time of stress and crisis.
plan for a crisis, and, therefore, are unpre-
spitalization contingencies they may face.
rue for elderly patients, who do not have
ems, such as family or friends, to help them
tion (Coulton et al., 1982). Other factors
cessful planning are lack of adequate post-
es, such as extended-care beds; limited
al staff in the necessary paperwork; and
al condition of the patient (Lurie, Pinskey,
chrager et al., 1978). Social workers tradi-
with patients and develop and advocate
ee access to high-quality care at all times
Lurie, Pinskey, and Tuzman, 1981).
harge patients early from acute-care hospi-
ct on the home care agencies that receive
(1982) studied the involvement of elderly
on long-term care. The factors that affect
evel of impairment, knowledge about long-
erceived freedom of choice, time available,
y power structure, compatibility of family
nion, social support, and patient's assert-
nd Coulton (1980) conducted a follow-up
harged from a hospital and found that a

The
may b
self-in
health
Adult

Sugge.
of Soc

HCI
reimbu
Howev
tion of
two to

Social

Curr
from a
degree
who is

Adjust

Proble

Loss
hearing
ment to

substantial number did not have their needs met, a reflection of the paucity of appropriate community services. The authors recommend follow-up of discharged patients to ensure that in-hospital planning is appropriate and that the plan is being implemented. They discovered that weaknesses exist in the continuing care system.

A boom in personnel needs in the area of gerontology and AIDS has been predicted. Other predictions are that hospital social work departments will downsize and that more social workers will move into home health care and nursing homes. There will also be an increase in third-party reimbursements for social workers, and more social workers will enter private practice.

GERIATRIC ASSESSMENT TEAM

Zink and Bissonnette (1990) describe a unique program in Boston that was started with funds from the Robert Wood Johnson Program. The program consists of a geriatric assessment team, composed of nurses and social workers, who provide assessment and services to high-risk elderly. To date, 200 elderly have benefitted from the program. The majority of assistance includes casework, help with alleviating unsafe or inappropriate housing and homelessness, and adjunct services. The program demonstrates the necessity of an interdisciplinary team approach to long-term treatment plans.

Pesznecker and Paquin (1982) recommend utilizing an interdisciplinary team practice with all geriatric home care clients. Zink (1987) gives us a tool for a holistic care assessment of older adults who are visited in the community. Lindner (1987) illustrates how home health care brings the hospital home because of prospective payment.

Goldstein (1989) predicts that physicians will be taking more active roles in the team approach, and house calls or home visits will return as ways of treating the elderly. Berkman and colleagues (1983) reports on the evaluation of an experimental, interdisciplinary geriatrics team responsible for total discharge planning of inpatients who are seventy-five years of age and older. Social work has the primary role of coordinating efforts.

This cluster also includes issues such as team development (Lee, 1980), administrative support and structure needed to create and use an interdisciplinary team conference (Clarke, Distasi, and Wallace, 1978), and interagency collaboration.

Other articles focus on themes such as professional identity, role overlap, and conflict (Lowe and Herranen, 1978), boundaries and areas of professional expertise, the team as reflective of systemic and patient care problems (Naisbitt, 1988), and ethical issues and decision making (Abramson, 1984).

POLICY ISSUES AND HEALTH CARE

The policy environment of health care organizations and health care practice is constantly in flux. Policies are affected by changing political priorities, the push and pull of various constituencies, the introduction of new ideas and technologies, and the advent of new health crises, such as AIDS. Several policy topics deserve special attention. For example:

1. Health care finance was the central issue of the 1970s, 1980s, and early 1990s. Among the factors that contributed to the rise in health care costs were growing elderly populations, introduction of new and expensive medical technologies, and expanding expectations regarding health care services. Those who paid for services, including government agencies, insurance companies such as Blue Cross/Blue Shield, and employers who provided costly health insurance as an employee benefit, were looking for ways to slow the inflationary spiral. No single issue had a greater effect on

the availability, quality, and nature of services than the issue of cost (Noble and Conley, 1982).
2. Medicare and Medicaid, including questions of entitlement, eligibility, and implementation (Davidson, 1982; Spring, 1981).
3. Long-term health care.
4. Primary health care.
5. Policies as they affect special populations, including children, the elderly, and the handicapped (Poole and Carlton, 1986).
6. Policies as they affect social work services, including the availability of funding to support social work services, education, and research resulting from decisions made in the public policy realm (Kane, 1985).
7. Policies as they affect social work services in home health care practice (NASW, 1991). Since the introduction of Medicare in the 1960s, home care services have become structured around a "medical model" or a "hospital service on wheels" (Olson and Mintun, 1990). Home health care, as a result, is losing much of its human services or family and community approaches.

FUTURE DIRECTIONS FOR HOME HEALTH CARE

Parker (1990) gives an interesting overview of what will assist the success of home health care in the future. The home health care industry is one of the fastest growing industries in the United States, and it shows little indication of slowing down. There are a variety of reasons for the rapid growth of home health care and the projected continued growth, including graying of the population, unique health and long-term care needs of the elderly, consumer preference, an increase in sophisticated medical technology, and changing federal policy.

As a group, the elderly are growing in number and proportion more rapidly than any other age group. The number of elderly persons (those over age sixty-five) increased from about three million in 1900 to twenty-eight million in 1984. If this trend continues, there will be thirty-two million elderly in the United States by the year 2000. In addition, the very old population (those over the age of eighty-five) is increasing even more rapidly. In 1980, there were two million persons over age eighty-five. That number is expected to increase to six million by the year 2000, and sixteen million by the year 2050. This is important because the elderly are the heaviest users of health and long-term care services in this country, including home health care.

According to Soldo and Manton (1985), the likelihood of chronic illness increases with age. Approximately 80 percent of the elderly in the community and nearly all those in long-term care facilities have at least one chronic condition. Functional dependencies, as measured by the capacity to perform basic activities of daily living, also increase with age. Direct need for assistance from another person in carrying out such basic functions as eating, bathing, and dressing increases from about one in ten (10 percent) for persons between sixty-five and seventy-four years of age to approximately 50 percent for those over age eighty-five (Soldo and Manton, 1985).

Functional dependency in the activities of daily living increases the need for and use of home health care. Studies have repeatedly shown that the elderly prefer to be treated and cared for at home rather than in an unfamiliar or institutional setting (Lerman, 1987; McAllister et al., 1986; McCann, 1987).

Campbell and Kennett (1987) gives some interesting insights into the future of home health care. Despite a demographic imperative that demonstrates a great demand for home care, a number of problems are looming, such as: the industry is not market driven; there is a competitive imbalance; administrators are engaged in crisis-oriented and reactive management; there is an absence of cohesive industry leadership; the sleeping giant—liability—affects everyone in home care; and the reimbursement crisis is only for those with limited vision. According to Campbell, "To be a visionary home care leader, an administrator should spend at least one hour per day contemplating the future of health care in his or her environment, make a commitment to quality, and plan for victory, not survival" (Campbell and Kennett, 1987).

Marketing techniques include physicians. Williams and Williams (1988) analyze the medical doctor as a client, and show home care agencies how to market to five types of physicians: high-tech, high-touch, care control, worry relief, and cannot be bothered. Some home health care agencies are already marketing to the families of clients and referral sources, and developing joint ventures and a special niche.

Griff and Lerman (1987) also predict that high-tech home care will grow rapidly. The development of sophisticated technologies facilitates earlier hospital discharge and increases the number of treatments given in the home. High-technology home therapy is one of the fastest growing segments of home health care, and is expected to transform the home into a primary site of clinical care in the twenty-first century (Griff and Lerman, 1987).

Parker (1990) addresses federal policy changes that spark home care growth. Changing federal policy since 1965 has had a marked effect on the growth of home health care utilization. The most significant federal policy changes include the Omnibus Budget Reconciliation Act (OBRA) in 1980 and the Tax Equity and Fiscal Responsibility Act (TEFRA) in 1982. OBRA 80 (PL 96-499) removed several major barriers to Medicare home health services. Limits on the number of visits in Parts A and B were eliminated, as were the three-day prior hospitalization and deductibles for Part B services.

Cabin (1986) discusses how the diagnostic related group (DRG) prospective payments system has been the major force in stimulating the home care industry. Hospitals are no longer reimbursed on the basis of reasonable cost, but on the basis of a predetermined capitated dollar amount per patient. Since hospitals are now paid a fixed dollar amount per patient, DRGs provide hospitals with the financial incentive to discharge patients from high-cost hospital environments to less costly settings. For this reason, DRGs are believed to have stimulated growth of the home care industry. Data show that hospital discharges into home care have increased 32 percent since the implementation of DRGs.

Many hospitals have developed home care agencies, which allow them to discharge their patients sooner, provide continuity of care, and keep patients and families within the hospital network.

According to the Health Care Financing Administration (1990), the number of hospital-based, Medicare-certified home care agencies grew from 579 in 1983 to 1,422 in 1987. This represents a 145 percent increase. The other largest growth was in proprietary (for-profit) agencies, which experienced an 84 percent increase.

MEDICARE STANDARDS FOR SOCIAL WORK PRACTICE IN HOME HEALTH CARE

Another large segment of the literature was related to the Medicare standards and social work services. In every aspect of health care, social work still plays a secondary role. We are still basing our entire health care delivery on a medical or acute care model rather than a preventative one. In home health care, social work does not even provide services unless it is ordered by the physician, and it is often even suggested by the RN who writes the order and then sends it to the physician to sign for their approval. In Medicaid-funded programs, social work service is not covered unless it is a mental health care-funded agency or in renal disease. In no other field except mental health care or renal disease is social work services mandated. Medicaid still does not reimburse for social work services in home care.

For many years, NASW has tried to get HCFA to grant skilled status to social work services, which would mandate that every patient receive at least an evaluation, but has failed. And now, with the new prospective payment system and the need to curtail costs, this does not seem likely to happen.

HEALTH CARE SPENDING AND REFORM

According to a study by HCFA (1992):

> By virtually all measures, U.S. health spending is the highest in the world. Over the past 10 years, whether in absolute dollar terms or relative to its GDP, U.S. health care expenditures have increased faster than spending in other countries, and the gap between the United States and other major industrialized countries has increased. The opportunity costs of U.S. health expenditure growth are the largest of the six major countries. Excess health care inflation in the United States exceeds excess health care inflation in other major countries. Health spending relative to GDP is increasing more rapidly in the United States than in other countries.

For health care reform to succeed, the United States must solve at least three problems that have been dealt with by other major industrialized countries. The poor and disadvantaged must be provided with health services, health insurance, or the financial means to purchase health insurance. For the nonpoor, a mechanism must be found to pool health risks while reforming private health insurance (e.g., having guaranteed issue, eliminating preexisting conditions, and nonrenewability clauses). Mechanisms must be found to control costs (Health Care Financing Administration, 1992).

GROUP WORK BY SOCIAL WORKERS

Group work has become a significant mode of social work intervention in health care settings. Much of the literature describes groups or group programs for patients and families who are coping with the psychological effects of a particular disease or life crisis, such as aging or institutionalization. Discussion of the special needs of a given population, the rationale for using a group approach, and the format or structure of the group are usually included.

Often, the literature focuses on a specific disease entity or life crisis. These include aging and institutionalization; Alzheimer's and related dementia (Shibbal-Champagne and Lipinska-Stachow, 1985-1986); bereavement (Roy and Sumpter, 1983); cancer (Roy and Sumpter, 1983); diabetes (Parry, 1980), physical disabilities (Evans et al., 1984); pulmonary disease (Foster and Mendel, 1979); renal disease (Roy, Flynn, and Atcherson, 1982); and visual impairments (Krausz, 1980).

Social workers working in home health care agencies are developing and leading many disease-focused groups. These include "I Can Cope Groups" for cancer patients, support groups for AIDS patients, and groups for those affected by pulmonary disease. There also are groups to stop smoking and to achieve weight loss.

In addition, there is extensive literature on the value and importance of caregiver support groups. These groups are mainly for support and education of caregivers who provide home-based health care to their spouses or loved ones.

DISEASE-SPECIFIC SOCIAL WORK PRACTICE

As the health care system becomes more specialized and high tech, the social work field also becomes more specialized. Schools of social work offer areas of study, such as gerontology, mental health, health, substance abuse, and family and children's services. But even within health care settings, there are specialties such as medicine, surgery, neurology, psychiatry, AIDS treatment, gerontology, oncology, renal disease, pediatrics, outpatient care, intensive care, and numerous others. Even in the home health care field, treatment is becoming more specialized.

Tamme (1985) found that home health care agencies need to be more attentive to abused and neglected adults being served by them. The author presents several key screening mechanisms to identify clients who are neglecting themselves or being neglected or abused by others. Also, most states have mandatory reporting laws for social workers, nurses, and other health care staff. Tamme stresses how social workers play an integral, necessary role in providing advocacy, support, casework, and linkage to services within the community.

Battle (1989) and Kruse and Wood (1989) give an excellent description of how to provide innovative and creative mental health services to homebound adults and the elderly. Both present a team-oriented approach utilizing a part-time psychiatrist, a full-time social worker, and a full-time nurse trained in psychiatric care. Clients are provided services and monitoring within their natural environments, and are encouraged to remain out of the hospital.

Gill (1991) conducts a case study on an interdisciplinary team serving stroke patients and their families in their homes. Social work services are provided to improve or maintain the socioemotional, functional, and physical health status of patients who have experienced strokes. Pendarvis and Grinnell (1980) call this approach "stroke rehabilitation teams," which are often developed within hospital settings.

Thoebaben and Woodward (1991) address the need for home care agencies to develop social work services to meet the psychosocial needs of homebound cardiac patients and their families. It is most important to assess and monitor the psychological well-being of patients who have experienced a myocardial infarction. This is often a neglected area of practice.

Frey and colleagues (1991) discuss the urgent need for home health care agencies to provide a team approach to meet the mental health needs of homebound AIDS patients.

Wilson (1989) conducted a grounded theory-based explanatory study of fifty-nine terminally ill patients being served by a hospice program in Wisconsin. The author also interviewed close kin and staff members. It was found that the hospice provided emphasis on mutual support, open communication, varied provisions for staff breaks, respite care, and general spiritual faith. The author also found very little turnover among hospice staff. Further research and policy ideas were generated.

Elian and Dean (1983) addressed another unique area, the social and mental health needs of patients living in the community who were afflicted with multiple sclerosis.

SOCIAL WORK PRACTICE
IN HOME HEALTH AGENCIES

A major implication of these findings is that if social workers in the United States are to play roles comparable to those in other countries, it is essential to have policies and services that incorporate a broader definition of dependency and impairment. Under the current, fragmented home care system, with its varied models and funding sources, it is difficult to foresee how such a definition can evolve without the active involvement of the social work profession.

According to Cox (1992), the home care programs of Manitoba, England, Sweden, and Norway illustrate how social work and sensitive social planning use an ecological perspective that could be incorporated into services. These programs are able to reduce nursing home admissions and enhance the quality of life of elderly people.

The programs differ in many significant aspects from those in the United States. For example, home care is universally offered on the basis of need, and need implies social dependency and frailty as well as medical need. Medical referrals or physician involvement in a case are not required for service. Throughout the programs, there is a focus on the interaction of the client with both social and environmental systems, and home care workers promote the competence of the individual to deal with these systems. Moreover, in several programs, the actual environment is frequently restructured to make it more responsive to the needs of the older person.

Cox (1992) also notes that description of programs in several countries illustrates the effectiveness of incorporating this perspective into services. The results include decreased rates of institutionalization, reduced costs, and more human and responsive systems of care. As new models of home health care evolve in the United States, social workers play key roles in their designs by emphasizing and improving their transactions within the community. Social workers are important change agents within their work environments.

The goal of social work services in home health care is to improve or maintain the social, emotional, functional, and physical health status of the patient, as well as to enhance the coping skills of the family or other caregiver system. Social work services make the critical difference between a patient completing a successful course of treatment and having to be rehospitalized or reinstitutionalized (NASW, 1991).

LITERATURE GAPS THE STUDY ADDRESSED

From an extensive review of the literature, it is apparent that our study focuses on a very specific area that has not been thoroughly explored. A number of journal articles from 1985 to the present have been reviewed. Most of the research and related literature discusses the clinical practice of social workers within home care, their impact on specific diseases and individuals, and how clients and families benefit. Another large segment of the literature focuses on early and effective discharge planning and how social work services play key roles. Numerous studies focus on the clinical benefit of social work services in medical settings. To date, there appears to be little research specifically on the behavioral aspects of home health agencies, staff and social workers, and their provision of social work services. The investigator decided to probe into the attitudes and beliefs of home health care staff and how factors affect the availability and utilization of social work services.

Factors affecting agency utilization of social work services appear to be a major area of inquiry missing in previous research. Our research focused on this gap, as well as why the researcher chose a grounded theory approach. The whole social work and home health care field is still a relatively new, increasing area of practice that has received very little attention in the health or social work arena. Most of the attention has focused on acute care, prospective payment, and the need for health care reform. Community-based care is now gaining more attention.

Chapter 9

Conclusions and Implications
for Future Applications and Research

The objective of this study was to explore home health care professionals' attitudes, perceptions, and beliefs about social workers and how they may affect the utilization of social work services.

This chapter summarizes the findings and conclusions from the research study and how they relate to future applications and research. The application of these findings in four major areas is discussed: social work practice in home care, home health care providers, social work education, and policy issues. The chapter concludes with implications for future research.

STUDY CONCLUSIONS

Several major conclusions can be drawn from the author's study and the writing of this book. Home care agencies have a working knowledge of what social workers do, which seems to fall into psychosocial assessments and community resource link-ages. Utilization of social work services is directly linked to staffing and the availability of the staff. Also, the higher the level of knowledge the agencies have, the higher the utilization will be. There is also a serious need for education and systematic knowledge about Medicare standards. Employing social work-ers, rather than contracting, seems to allow better utilization.

Home health care agencies also have found it more difficult to recruit licensed independent social workers. In some states, social workers licensed at the bachelor's level cannot practice in home health care without supervision. Long-term services such as transportation, chore services, and personal care are a serious community need. Physicians and the general public still lack knowledge of social work services. The notion that all social workers work for the "welfare" system is still prevalent. Medicaid still does not reimburse for social work services.

Some personality factors also allow higher utilization, including flexibility, the ability to act independently, an outgoing personality, a high level of maturity, and the ability to enter unpredictable situations. Also, social workers must be more assertive in home care agencies to be noticed, to receive referrals, and to be considered part of the team.

Home care agencies need to develop more educational programs in home health and social work areas, such as workshops, seminars, and forming alliances with schools of social work. There is a desperate need for schools of social work to incorporate home health care and community practice into their curriculums. Students should be encouraged to complete their field placements in home health care agencies.

And last, Medicare still does not pay for social work services in home health care. We still do not have a long-term strategy. Long-term services are still not available for numerous individuals.

It is recommended that the study be replicated in other settings in order to generalize the findings. Of additional importance is the need to conduct a study with Medicare regulatory agencies regarding their understanding of the standards related to social work services and home health care.

Looking Toward the Future

The Balanced Budget Act of 1997 established a new reimbursement system for home health care with cost-based, reduced limits and a per-beneficiary cap of approximately $3,500 per Medicare beneficiary. This new system, which takes the industry toward a prospective pay model, has had far-reaching, drastic effects. It is now believed that this system has seriously jeopardized patients' access to home health care benefits, especially for therapies such as social work, physical therapy, and occupational therapy. Agencies must manage their utilization of services and many are not ordering these more expensive services. Therefore, fewer services are being delivered to the nation's disabled and the elderly, especially those with complex medical and psychosocial needs.

The BBA was designed to stem the growth of the Medicare home health benefit by reducing spending over a five-year period by $16.1 billion. Instead, the cuts have been more than $47 billion—more than 300 percent more than intended (National Association of Home Care, 1999). Unfortunately, this has been done at the expense of many frail elderly and disabled patients who desperately need the services to lead higher-quality lives, to continue living in the community, and to stay out of costly institutions.

Congress is currently supportive of reform measures and the National Association of Home Care is the leader in looking at ways to optimize Medicare savings while maintaining medically necessary services. No one really knows what the future holds for home health care services, but as our elderly population continues to grow, it must remain a viable option and a less costly one than institutional care.

Social workers and other health care professionals must continue to advocate for these services to remain available and accessible to our clients.

Home health care is now experiencing drastic cuts, new regulations and standards, extensive fraud and abuse, and turmoil. Many agencies across the country have either closed, merged, or been purchased by larger systems.

Because of the need to control costs, Medicare introduced a prospective pay system beginning in 1997, which has already caused drastic cuts in home health care visits in every discipline, including social work.

Home health care is now experiencing the same changes observed in hospitals in the 1980s with the DRG system. The financial incentives and profit margins for home health agencies will never be the same. It is my hope, though, that the needs of clients are not lost during this major crisis, and, especially, that social work will remain a vital part of the treatment team.

Appendix A

Recruitment Letter
for Research Participants

Date

Attention: Director
Home Health Care Agency
Address

As you already know, home health care is a fast-growing industry and will continue to grow as more people age and hospital discharges occur early in a patient's healing process.

I have been working in home care for the last six years as a social work service provider. I am also a PhD student and am very interested in the area of social work service utilization within home care agencies for my dissertation. I am writing you to express my sincere interest in having your agency participate in this research study. My study focuses on home health agency staff attitudes, beliefs, perceptions, and utilization of social work staff. I am also interested in a combination of urban, rural, and suburban based agencies. I want a variety of agencies having different Medicare Intermediaries. I am particularly interested in looking at Medicare standards and how these might impact what I'm researching.

The actual study will consist of two interviews within each agency. There will be one interview lasting about one and a half hours with the director of the agency and the director of nursing and/or quality assurance. The second interview will consist of a focus group made up of clinical staff consisting of RN case managers, OTs, PTs, speech therapists, and home health aides. This interview will last one and a half to two hours and will be audiotaped. In each interview, the researcher will ask general, open-ended questions about the subject area. This will encourage open discussion and an emerging theory.

The researcher will need to review some written policies, procedures, visits, philosophy, and other materials related to social work service. Each agency will be analyzed and the results written as a separate case study. All information will be strictly confidential. The study is to promote more scholarly knowledge within the home health care field and promote published articles in nursing and social work journals. If you agree to be a participant in the study, please return the enclosed, addressed, stamped postcard. Thank you very much.

Sincerely,

Ruth Ann Goode

Appendix B

Interview Questions

QUESTIONS USED FOR CLINICAL FOCUS GROUP INTERVIEWS

1. What do social workers in home care perform?

2. Do you refer your patients for medical social work services?

3. What is your understanding of Medicare's guidelines for social work services?

4. Do you find any social work staff problems in recruitment, retention, training, credentials, etc.?

5. Obstacles in providing social work services?

6. What can be done to assist home care agencies in providing social work services?

7. How do you assess a patient's need for social work services?

8. Do you believe your social work services are being utilized appropriately?

9. What service gaps do you see in your community after social workers assess your patients?

10. Should social work be an independent, skilled, reimbursable service similar to nursing and physical or speech therapy?

11. Any further ideas or suggestions?

QUESTIONS USED FOR ADMINISTRATIVE INTERVIEWS

1. What do you believe social workers in home care do?

2. What is your understanding of Medicare's guidelines for social work and reimbursement?

3. How many visits per patient does your intermediary agency allow?

4. Do you believe Medicare's rules are sufficient?

5. Do you find any social work personnel shortages in the home health field?

6. Any suggestions related to staffing?

7. Do you believe your utilization of social work visits is sufficient for the number of patients you serve?

8. What do you think could be done to assist home care agencies in providing social work services?

Appendix C

Consent Form

THE UTILIZATION OF SOCIAL WORK IN HOME HEALTH CARE AGENCIES

You are invited to be in a research study that focuses on home health care staffs' attitudes, perceptions, beliefs, and utilization of social workers and their services. You were selected as a possible participant because of your voluntary interest. We ask that you read this form and ask any questions you may have before agreeing to be in the study.

This study is being conducted by: Walden University.

Background Information

The purpose of the study is to examine the beliefs, perceptions, and attitudes of home health care staff about social workers and their services. Two interviews will take place within twelve home care agencies. One will be with the administrator and director of nursing, and the other will be a focus group interview with ten to twelve clinical staff members, OTs, PTs, and RNs. A general topical outline will be used as questions to promote open discussion. The researcher will listen, take notes, and analyze findings. New theory development is the focus. Also, the researcher wants to review some administration records related to agencies' philosophy, mission, policies, procedures, and statistics related to social work visits. Information will be confidential, known only to the researcher.

New scholarly knowledge within the home health care field will be gained.

Procedures

1. You will be a participant in a focus group made up of clinical staff within your own agency.
2. The group of ten to twelve participants will only meet once for one and a half to two hours.
3. The participants will answer and discuss leading questions of inquiry by the researcher.
4. The focus group will be audiotape recorded so that data and feedback can be analyzed.
5. Participation is fully voluntary.
6. You might wish to write down, before the group meets, your ideas and thoughts about social workers and home care.

Compensation

You will receive no payment. The principal investigator will provide a lunch for the participants at each agency to express thanks and appreciation.

Confidentiality

The records of this study will be kept private. In any sort of report we might publish, we will not include any information that will make it possible to identify a subject. Research records will be kept in a locked file; only the researchers will have access to the records. An audiotape will be recorded of each focus group, which only the principal investigator will have access to. The tapes will be erased three months later.

Voluntary Nature of the Study

Your decision whether to participate will not affect your current or future relations with the University. If you decide to participate, you are free to withdraw at any time without affecting those relationships.

Contacts and Questions

The researchers conducting this study are PhD student Ruth Ann Goode and Dr. Marcia Steinhauer. You may ask any questions you have now. If you have questions later, you may contact them. You will be given a copy of this form to keep for your records.

Statement of Consent

I have read the above information. I have asked questions and received answers. I consent to participate in the study.

Signature: _____ Date: _____

Signature of Investigator: _____ Date: _____

Appendix D

Home Health Agencies
Who Participated in the Study

First American Home Care, Columbus, Ohio

Professional Nursing Service, Cuyahoga Falls, Ohio

Nurses House Calls, Akron, Ohio

Health Care in Your Home, Canton, Ohio

Nursefinders of Cleveland and Akron, Shaker Heights, Ohio

American Professional Home Health, Inc., Cleveland, Ohio

University Mednet Home Care, Inc., Eastlake, Ohio

Ashtabula Regional Home Health Services, Ashtabula, Ohio

Interim Health Care, Toledo, Ohio

Visiting Nurse Association, Youngstown, Ohio

TRI-County Home Nurses, Wadsworth, Ohio

Enriched Living, Cincinnati, Ohio

Appendix E

Documentation System for Social Workers

PHYSICIAN ORDERS

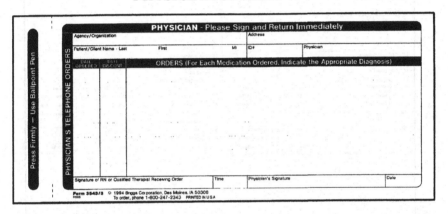

Source: Reprinted with permission of Briggs Corporation, Des Moines, Iowa, (800) 247-2343.

HOME HEALTH CERTIFICATION
AND PLAN OF CARE

Department of Health and Human Services Health Care Financing Administration					Form Approved OMB No. 0938-0357
		HOME HEALTH CERTIFICATION AND PLAN OF CARE			
1. Patient's HI Claim No.	2. Start Of Care Date	3. Certification Period From: To:		4. Medical Record No.	5. Provider No.
6. Patient's Name and Address			7. Provider's Name, Address and Telephone Number		
8. Date of Birth		9. Sex ☐ M ☐ F	10. Medications: Dose/Frequency/Route (N)ew (C)hanged		
11 ICD-9-CM	Principal Diagnosis	Date			
12. ICD-9-CM	Surgical Procedure	Date			
13. ICD-9-CM	Other Pertinent Diagnoses	Date			
14. DME and Supplies			15. Safety Measures.		
16. Nutritional Req.			17. Allergies:		

18.A. Functional Limitations

1 ☐ Amputation	5 ☐ Paralysis	9 ☐ Legally Blind
2 ☐ Bowel/Bladder (Incontinence)	6 ☐ Endurance	A ☐ Dyspnea With Minimal Exertion
3 ☐ Contracture	7 ☐ Ambulation	B ☐ Other (Specify)
4 ☐ Hearing	8 ☐ Speech	

18.B. Activities Permitted

1 ☐ Complete Bedrest	6 ☐ Partial Weight Bearing	A ☐ Wheelchair
2 ☐ Bedrest BRP	7 ☐ Independent At Home	B ☐ Walker
3 ☐ Up As Tolerated	8 ☐ Crutches	C ☐ No Restrictions
4 ☐ Transfer Bed/Chair	9 ☐ Cane	D ☐ Other (Specify)
5 ☐ Exercises Prescribed		

19. Mental Status:

| 1 ☐ Oriented | 3 ☐ Forgetful | 5 ☐ Disoriented | 7 ☐ Agitated |
| 2 ☐ Comatose | 4 ☐ Depressed | 6 ☐ Lethargic | 8 ☐ Other |

20. Prognosis: 1 ☐ Poor   2 ☐ Guarded   3 ☐ Fair   4 ☐ Good   5 ☐ Excellent

21. Orders for Discipline and Treatments (Specify Amount/Frequency/Duration)

22. Goals/Rehabilitation Potential/Discharge Plans

23. Nurse's Signature and Date of Verbal SOC Where Applicable:	25. Date HHA Received Signed POT
24. Physician's Name and Address	26. I certify/recertify that this patient is confined to his/her home and needs intermittent skilled nursing care, physical therapy and/or speech therapy or continues to need occupational therapy. The patient is under my care, and I have authorized the services on this plan of care and will periodically review the plan.
27. Attending Physician's Signature and Date Signed	28. Anyone who misrepresents, falsifies, or conceals essential information required for payment of Federal funds may be subject to fine, imprisonment, or civil penalty under applicable Federal laws.
Form 3488N/4P BRIGGS, Des Moines, IA 50306 (800) 247-2343 PRINTED IN U.S.A.	**PROVIDER** Form HCFA-485 (C-4) (02-94) (Print Aligned)

Source: Reprinted with permission of Briggs Corporation, Des Moines, Iowa, (800) 247-2343.

ADDENDUM: MEDICAL UPDATE

Department of Health and Human Services Health Care Financing Administration				Form Approved OMB No. 0938-0357	
ADDENDUM TO:		☐ **PLAN OF TREATMENT**	☐ **MEDICAL UPDATE**		
1. Patient's HI Claim No.	2. SOC Date	3. Certification Period From: To:	4. Medical Record No.	5. Provider No.	
6. Patient's Name		7. Provider Name			

8. Item
   No.

9. Signature of Physician   10. Date

11. Optional Name/Signature of Nurse/Therapist   12. Date

Source: Reprinted with permission of Briggs Corporation, Des Moines, Iowa, (800) 247-2343.

INTERDISCIPLINARY REFERRAL

INTERDISCIPLINARY REFERRAL

CARE MANAGER _____

DATE OF REFERRAL ____/____/____

USE THE COMMENTS AREA TO FURTHER EXPLAIN CHECKED ITEMS AND/OR TO PROVIDE ADDITIONAL PERTINENT INFORMATION

PHYSICAL THERAPY

REASON FOR REFERRAL: ☐ Home safety evaluation   ☐ ADL or ambulation   ☐ Teach caregiver/spouse
☐ Other (specify)_____

COMMENTS: _____

SHOULD BE SEEN WITHIN _____ DAYS/WEEKS   ORDERED/RECOMMENDED FREQUENCY _____

OCCUPATIONAL THERAPY

REASON FOR REFERRAL:
☐ UE sensorimotor program   ☐ Joint protection
☐ Environmental adaptation   ☐ Cognitive/Perceptual adaptation   ☐ COPD program
☐ Positioning equipment   ☐ Custom equipment/accessories   ☐ Hand splints & therapy
☐ Modified self-care   ☐ Home management & functional mobility   ☐ Energy conservation
☐ Work simplification   ☐ Other (specify)_____

COMMENTS: _____

SHOULD BE SEEN WITHIN _____ DAYS/WEEKS   ORDERED/RECOMMENDED FREQUENCY _____

SPEECH/LANGUAGE PATHOLOGY

REASON FOR REFERRAL: ☐ Swallowing problems   .   ☐ Communication assistance   ☐ Slurred speech   ☐ Expression
☐ Other (specify)_____

COMMENTS: _____

SHOULD BE SEEN WITHIN _____ DAYS/WEEKS   ORDERED/RECOMMENDED FREQUENCY _____

SOCIAL SERVICE

REASON FOR REFERRAL: ☐ Identified social problem that is impeding effective implementation of POC (specify below)
☐ Community resources   ☐ Placement   ☐ Counseling/Psychosocial problem(s)   ☐ Needs/Home assessment
☐ Other (specify)_____

COMMENTS: _____

SHOULD BE SEEN WITHIN _____ DAYS/WEEKS   ORDERED/RECOMMENDED FREQUENCY _____

SKILLED NURSING

REASON FOR REFERRAL: ☐ Evaluation   ☐ Skin assessment   ☐ CVR assessment   ☐ Medication program
☐ Suture removal   ☐ Bladder/Bowel care   ☐ Other (specify)_____

COMMENTS: _____

SHOULD BE SEEN WITHIN _____ DAYS/WEEKS   ORDERED/RECOMMENDED FREQUENCY _____

PHYSICIAN _____   PHONE _____

VERBAL ORDER OBTAINED FROM MD FOR REFERRAL TO: ☐ SN   ☐ Aide   ☐ PT   ☐ OT   ☐ SLP   ☐ MSW   ☐ Dietary
☐ Other (specify)_____

OTHER DISCIPLINES INVOLVED IN CARE: ☐ SN   ☐ Aide   ☐ PT   ☐ OT   ☐ SLP   ☐ MSW   ☐ Dietary
☐ Other (specify)_____

PERSON COMPLETING FORM
SIGNATURE/TITLE _____   DATE ____/____/____

PART 1 — Clinical Record   PART 2 — Discipline Referred To   PART 3 — Care Coordinator

PATIENT/CLIENT NAME — Last, First, Middle Initial   ID #

Form 3582/3P   © 1994 Briggs Corporation, Des Moines, IA 50306   **INTERDISCIPLINARY REFERRAL**
To order, phone 1-800-247-2343   PRINTED IN USA

Source: Reprinted with permission of Briggs Corporation, Des Moines, Iowa, (800) 247-2343.

MEDICAL SOCIAL SERVICES EVALUATION

MEDICAL SOCIAL SERVICES EVALUATION

DATE OF SERVICE ___ / ___ / ___

TIME IN ___   OUT ___

HOMEBOUND REASON: ☐ Needs assistance for all activities   ☐ Residual weakness
☐ Requires assistance to ambulate   ☐ Confusion, unable to go out of home alone
☐ Unable to safely leave home unassisted   ☐ Severe SOB, SOB upon exertion
☐ Dependent upon adaptive device(s)   ☐ Medical restrictions
☐ Other (specify) ___

TYPE OF EVALUATION
☐ Initial   ☐ Interim   ☐ Final
SOC DATE ___ / ___ / ___
(If Initial Evaluation, complete Medical Social Services Care Plan, for 3598/3P)

ORDERS FOR EVALUATION ONLY? ☐ Yes   ☐ No   If no, orders are ___

PERTINENT BACKGROUND INFORMATION

MEDICAL DIAGNOSIS/PROBLEM ___ **ONSET** ___ / ___ / ___

PRIOR LEVEL OF ADL STATUS ___

PRIOR PERTINENT MEDICAL/SOCIAL HISTORY ___

MEDICAL SOCIAL SERVICES ASSESSMENT

PSYCHOSOCIAL (Describe mental status, coping ability, attitude, safety prognosis and implications, etc.) ___

CURRENT LIVING SITUATION/SUPPORT SYSTEM (Describe relationships/communications/interactions with family/caregiver/ significant other, etc.) ___

HEALTH FACTORS (Describe those factors that impede the POC from being effectively implemented, i.e., vision, hearing, nutrition, etc.) ___

ENVIRONMENTAL FACTORS (Describe those factors that impede the POC from being effectively implemented, i.e., transportation, safety, etc.) ___

FINANCIAL STATUS (Describe resources, income, assets/expenses, etc. that impede the POC from being effectively implemented.) ___

SIGNATURE/DATE

Complete TIME OUT (above) prior to signing below.

MEDICAL SOCIAL WORKER SIGNATURE/TITLE ___ **DATE** ___ / ___ / ___

PART 1 — Clinical Record	PART 2 — MSS	PART 3 — Care Coordination
PATIENT/CLIENT NAME — Last, First, Middle Initial		ID#

Form 3597/3P   © 1994 Briggs Corporation, Des Moines, IA 50306
To order, phone 1-800-247-2343   PRINTED IN U.S.A.

MEDICAL SOCIAL SERVICES EVALUATION

MEDICAL SOCIAL SERVICES

Source: Reprinted with permission of Briggs Corporation, Des Moines, Iowa, (800) 247-2343.

CARE SUMMARY

CARE SUMMARY

☐ Transfer/Referral
☐ Recert. Summary/Order Renewal
☐ Discharge Summary

PATIENT/CLIENT_____ ID#_____
ADDRESS _____
PHONE _____
SOC ___/___/___ Most Recent ___/___/___ (If applicable) Last Date of Service ___/___/___
Recert.

PHYSICIAN _____
☐ Notified ___/___/___
☐ POT 485 Attached for Signature
☐ Copy Sent ___/___/___

DISCIPLINES INVOLVED
☐ SN   ☐ PT   ☐ SLP
☐ HHA   ☐ OT   ☐ MSW
☐ Other _____
☐ Other _____

SUMMARY

THIS SUMMARY AREA MUST BE COMPLETED IN ALL CASES

REASON FOR ADMISSION (describe condition) _____

SUMMARY OF CARE (to date) _____

DISCHARGE

If Discharge Summary checked in upper right, indicate reason and date below.

☐ Patient/Client-centered goals achieved ___/___/___
☐ Patient/Client expired ___/___/___
☐ Geographic relocation ___/___/___
☐ Transfer/Admit to other agency/organization/facility (Complete Transfer/Referral section below.) ___/___/___
☐ Patient/Client refused further care ___/___/___
☐ No longer home bound ___/___/___
☐ Agency/Organization decision ___/___/___
Explain: _____

☐ Patient/Client/Family request ___/___/___
☐ Physician request ___/___/___
☐ Repeatedly not home/not found ___/___/___
☐ Patient/Client refused to accept care/treatments as ordered ___/___/___
☐ Persistent noncompliance with POC ___/___/___
☐ Failure to maintain services of an attending physician ___/___/___
☐ Other (specify)_____ ___/___/___

CONDITION AT DISCHARGE (describe) _____

DISCHARGE PLANNING (specify future follow-up, referrals, etc.)_____

Written instructions given to patient/client/caregiver: ☐ Yes ☐ No, explain _____
Patient/Client/Caregiver demonstrates understanding of instructions: ☐ Yes ☐ No, explain _____

TRANSFER/REFERRAL

UNIQUE NEEDS AND/OR BIO-PSYCHOSOCIAL PROBLEMS (specify) _____

Medication information attached   ☐ Yes   ☐ No
Advance directive exists   ☐ Yes   ☐ No   Copy attached   ☐ Yes   ☐ No

Signature/Title: _____ Date: ___/___/___

PART 1 — Clinical Record   PART 2 — Physician or Transfer Organization   PART 3 — Care Coordination

PATIENT/CLIENT NAME — Last, First, Middle Initial   ID#

CARE SUMMARY

Source: Reprinted with permission of Briggs Corporation, Des Moines, Iowa, (800) 247-2343.

DAILY ACTIVITY LOG

DAILY ACTIVITY LOG

DATE OF SERVICE ____ / ____ / ____

EMPLOYEE NAME _____ I.D.# _____

☐ RN ☐ LPN/LVN ☐ AIDE ☐ PT ☐ LPTA ☐ OT ☐ COTA ☐ SLP ☐ MSW ☐ BSW ☐ OTHER (specify) _____

PATIENT/CLIENT NAME AND ID#		VISIT CODE	START TIME	END TIME	ACTUAL VISIT TIME	NON-VISIT TIME		MILEAGE			BILLABLE SUPPLIES USED
NAME—Last, First	ID#					HOURS	CODE	START	END	MILES	

VISIT CODES		NON-VISIT CODES			
A - Admit	R - Refused Svc.	T - Travel Time	SM - Staff Meeting		
AE - Admin./Eval. Visit Only	⊖ - Not Home	I - Inservice	S - Seminar		
RV - Revisit	__ - __	CC - Care Conference	__ - __		
AS - Aide Super. Only	__ - __	OC - On Call	__ - __		
ASR - Aide Super. and RV	__ - __	O - Orientation	__ - __		

TOTAL MILES _____

LESS PERSONAL MILES _____

REIMBURSABLE MILES _____

PART 1 — Supervisor   PART 2 — Business Office/Data Processing   PART 3 — Individual Staff Member

DAILY ACTIVITY LOG

Form 3644/3P   © 1994 Briggs Corporation, Des Moines, IA 50306
To order, phone 1-800-247-2343 PRINTED IN U.S.A.

Source: Reprinted with permission of Briggs Corporation, Des Moines, Iowa, (800) 247-2343.

MEDICAL SOCIAL SERVICES CARE PLAN

MEDICAL SOCIAL SERVICES CARE PLAN

SOC DATE ___/___/___

REASON FOR VISIT/PROBLEM

MEDICAL SOCIAL SERVICES TREATMENT PLAN

PATIENT/CLIENT DESIRED OUTCOMES	SHORT TERM OUTCOMES	Time Frame	LONG TERM OUTCOMES	Time Frame

PLAN OF CARE

Assessment of social and emotional factors (E1)	Arrange transportation for medical appointments	Services to family member(s)/caregiver(s)
Counseling for long-range planning and decision making (E2)	Emotional support to patient/client/family	
Community resource planning (E3)	Financial resource information	Referral to support group(s)/ community resource(s) (specify)
Short term therapy (E4)	Arrangement of meal services	
Identify eligibility for services/benefits	Initiate abuse reporting mechanism	
Initiate counseling	Initiate referral to personal emergency response system	
Nursing home placement assistance	Teach self-management skills	Other:
Alternate living arrangements	Crisis intervention	

COMMENTS/ADDITIONAL INFORMATION _____

PATIENT/CLIENT/CAREGIVER RESPONSE TO PLAN OF CARE _____

SUMMARY

GOALS ACHIEVED? ☐ Yes ☐ No
Specify _____

APPROXIMATE NEXT VISIT DATE ___/___/___
PLAN FOR NEXT VISIT _____

REFERRALS COMPLETED? ☐ Yes ☐ No
Specify _____

DISCHARGE DISCUSSED WITH: ☐ Patient/Client/Family
☐ Care Manager ☐ Physician ☐ Other_____
DISCHARGE INSTRUCTIONS GIVEN TO PATIENT/CLIENT/
FAMILY? ☐ No ☐ Yes, specify_____

CARE COORDINATION: ☐ Care Manager, date ___/___/___
☐ Physician, date ___/___/___ ☐ Other (specify)_____

SIGNATURES/DATES

X _____ ___/___/___   X _____ ___/___/___
Patient/Client/Caregiver (if applicable) Date   Medical Social Worker (signature/title)   Date

PART 1 — Clinical Record   PART 2 — MSS   PART 3 — Care Coordination

PATIENT/CLIENT NAME — Last, First, Middle Initial   ID#

Form 3688/3P   © 1994 Briggs Corporation, Des Moines, IA 50306
3890   To order, phone 1-800-247-2343 PRINTED IN U.S.A.

MEDICAL SOCIAL SERVICES CARE PLAN

MEDICAL SOCIAL SERVICES

Source: Reprinted with permission of Briggs Corporation, Des Moines, Iowa, (800) 247-2343.

MEDICAL SOCIAL SERVICES REVISIT NOTE

MEDICAL SOCIAL SERVICES REVISIT NOTE

DATE OF VISIT ___/___/___

TIME IN _____ TIME OUT_____

MEDICAL SOCIAL SERVICES

HOMEBOUND REASON: ☐ Needs assistance for all activities ☐ Residual weakness
☐ Requires assistance to ambulate ☐ Confusion, unable to go out of home alone
☐ Unable to safely leave home unassisted ☐ Severe SOB, SOB upon exertion
☐ Dependent upon adaptive device(s) ☐ Medical restrictions
☐ Other (specify) _____

REASON FOR VISIT/PROBLEM _____

ASSESSMENT/OBSERVATION (Current situation, i.e., psychosocial, physical condition, environment, etc.)

MEDICAL SOCIAL SERVICES INTERVENTIONS (If applicable, mark with "X".)

Assessment of social and emotional factors (E1)	Arrange transportation for medical appointments	Services to family member(s)/caregiver(s)
Counseling for long-range planning and decision making (E2)	Emotional support to patient/client/family	
	Financial resource information	Referral to support group(s)/ community resource(s) (specify)
Community resource planning (E3)	Arrangement of meal services	
Short-term therapy (E4)	Initiate abuse reporting mechanism	
Identify eligibility for services/benefits	Initiate referral to personal emergency response system	
Initiate counseling		
Nursing home placement assistant	Teach self-management skills	Other:
Alternate living arrangements	Crisis intervention	

ANALYSIS OF FINDINGS/INTERVENTIONS/INSTRUCTIONS _____

EVALUATION AND PATIENT/CLIENT/CAREGIVER RESPONSE _____

SUMMARY

GOALS ACHIEVED? ☐ Yes ☐ No
Specify _____

APPROXIMATE NEXT VISIT DATE ___/___/___
PLAN FOR NEXT VISIT _____

REFERRALS COMPLETED? ☐ Yes ☐ No
Specify _____

DISCHARGE DISCUSSED WITH: ☐ Patient/Client/Family
☐ Care Manager ☐ Physician ☐ Other _____
DISCHARGE INSTRUCTIONS GIVEN TO PATIENT/CLIENT/ FAMILY? ☐ No ☐ Yes, specify _____

CARE COORDINATION: ☐ Care Manager, date ___/___/___
☐ Physician, date ___/___/___ ☐ Other (specify) _____

SIGNATURES/DATES:

X _____ Date ___/___/___
Patient/Client/Caregiver (if applicable)

X _____ Date ___/___/___
Medical Social Worker (Signature/title)

PART 1 — Clinical Record   PART 2 — MSS   PART 3 — Care Coordination

PATIENT/CLIENT NAME — Last, First, Middle Initial   ID*

Form 3581/3P © 1994 Briggs Corporation, Des Moines, IA 50306
To order, phone 1-800-247-2343 PRINTED IN USA

MEDICAL SOCIAL SERVICES REVISIT NOTE

VISIT/CALENDAR WORKSHEET

**PRESCRIBED VISITS
CALENDAR WORKSHEET**

DISC.	FREQ/WKS	FREQ/WKS	FREQ/WKS	FREQ/WKS	FREQ/WKS
SN					
HHA					
PT					
OT					
SLP					
MSS					

SOC DATE ___/___/___

WEEK NO.	FILL IN DAYS OF WEEK — BEGIN WITH SOC DATE/DAY						
1							
2							
3							
4							
5							
6							
7							
8							
9							

PATIENT/CLIENT NAME - Last, First, Middle Initial   ID/

Form 3840P   © 1994 Briggs Corporation, Des Moines, IA 50306
rev.   To order, phone 1-800-247-2343 PRINTED IN U.S.A.   **PRESCRIBED VISITS CALENDAR WORKSHEET**

Source: Reprinted with permission of Briggs Corporation, Des Moines, Iowa, (800) 247-2343.

CARE COORDINATION NOTE

CARE COORDINATION NOTE

COORDINATION OF CARE WITH: ☐ Physician ☐ RN/LPN/LVN ☐ Aide ☐ PT/LPTA ☐ OT/COTA ☐ SLP ☐ MSS
☐ Pharmacist ☐ Dietitian ☐ HME ☐ Resp. Therapist ☐ Community Resource ☐ Other _____

COMMUNICATED VIA: ☐ Phone ☐ Direct ☐ Mail ☐ Fax ☐ Other _____

Area/Problem Discussed

_____
_____
_____
_____
_____
_____
_____

Resolution/Follow-Up

_____
_____
_____
_____

PERSON COMPLETING FORM:
Signature/Title _____ Date ___/___/___ Time _____

PART 1 — Clinical Record   PARTS 2 and 3 — Care Coordination

PATIENT/CLIENT NAME — Last, First, Middle Initial   ID#

Form 3677/3 © 1994 Briggs Corporation, Des Moines, IA 50306   **CARE COORDINATION NOTE**
To order, phone 1-800-247-2343 PRINTED IN U S A

Source: Reprinted with permission of Briggs Corporation, Des Moines, Iowa, (800) 247-2343.

Glossary

The following terms have been used throughout this book and are defined here. The Ohio Council of Home Care *Resource Guide* (1997) was used for reference.

Activities of daily living (ADL): A measure that describes the presence and severity of disability among the elderly.

Case management: An administrative service that directs client movement through a series of phased involvements with the health and social services delivery system with the goal of increasing the quality and cost effectiveness of care.

Discharge planning: Generally, hospital-based programs that coordinate continuing or follow-up care for a patient during hospitalization and after his or her discharge from the hospital.

Home health aide: Also known as home care aide; an individual who may have received training to provide personal care. Unless a home health aide is certified, he or she may not have provided personal care under a plan of care prescribed by a physician.

Home visit: A significant contact with or on behalf of a patient in the patient's place of residence.

Homemaker service: A person who performs general household duties, such as cooking, cleaning, child care, and shopping. A homemaker is not trained to provide personal care.

Hospice: A coordinated program of palliative and supportive care for individuals who experience terminal illness; an interdisciplinary team of professionals and volunteers providing services in the patient's residence, or in an inpatient setting, during an illness or period of bereavement.

Intermittent care: Home health care services provided on an episodic basis.

Medicaid: National health care program created by Title XIX of the Social Security Act and administered by the states to provide health care to indigent and medically indigent persons of all ages.

Medical social work services: Services provided by a trained social worker, which include psychosocial assessment, counseling, and decision making, long-term planning, and linkage to community resources.

Medicare: National medical insurance program created by Title XVIII of the Social Security Act that provides health and medical insurance for persons over age sixty-five and others eligible for Social Security benefits.

Occupational therapy: Occupational therapy (OT) is needed if a patient has suffered an injury or illness. It assists patients in developing perceptual motor skills and in performing activities of daily living, such as dressing, eating, and cooking. Occupational Therapists are registered by the American Occupational Therapy Association.

Personal care: Activities such as bathing, dressing, grooming, and caring for hair, nails, and oral hygiene, which are needed to facilitate treatment or prevent deterioration of health; also assistance with feeding, elimination, ambulation, transfers, and changing positions in bed.

Physical therapy: Physical therapy is needed if a patient has suffered an injury or illness that has affected motor skills or functions. It assists patients in gaining endurance, gait training, ambulation, exercise, and restoration of activities.

Skilled nursing: Activities that require the skills of a registered nurse or licensed practical nurse, including assessment, education, and administration of medications and treatments.

References

Abramson, M. (1984). Collective responsibility in interdisciplinary collaboration: An ethical perspective for social workers. *Social Work, 10*(1), 35-44.

Battle, M. G. (1989). Social work mental health services and the long-term care continuum. *Gerontology and Geriatrics Education, 9*(3), 49-59.

Ben-Sira, Z. and Szyf, M. (1992). Status inequality in the nurse-social worker collaboration in hospitals. *Journal of Social Science Medicine, 34*(4), 365-374.

Berkman, B., Campion, E., Swaggerty, G., and Goldman, M. (1983). Geriatric consultation team: Alternative approach to social work discharge planning. *Journal of Gerontological Social Work, 5*(3), 77-88.

Bernstein, B. (1980). Legal needs of the ill: The social worker role in an interdisciplinary team. *Health and Social Work, 5*(3), 68-72.

Bjorkhem, K., Olsson, A., Hallberg, I. R., and Norberg, A. (1992). Caregivers' experience of providing care for demented persons living at home. *Scandinavian Journal of Primary Health Care, 10*(1), 53-59.

Cabin, W. D. (1986). *A primer on managed care for the home care industry.* Totowa, NJ: Home Health Associates.

Campbell, L. and Kennett, M. O. (1987). *Home care and the future.* Englewood, CO: Health-Net Publications.

Capra, R. (1982). *The turning point.* New York: Simon and Schuster.

Chenitz, C. and Swanson, J. (1986). *From practice to grounded theory.* Menlo Park, CA: Addison-Wesley.

Clarke, T. R., Distasi, W. L., and Wallace, C. (1978). Developing a multi-disciplinary conference. *Health and Social Work, 3*(1), 166-174.

Coulton, C., Dunkle, R., Goode, R., and Mackintosh, J. (1982). Discharge planning and decision making. *Health and Social Work, 7*(4), 253-261.

Cox, C. (1992). Expanding social work's role in home care: An ecological perspective. *Social Work, 37*(2), 179-183.

Davidson, S. (1982). Medicaid. In D. Lum (Ed.), *Social work and health care policy* (pp. 57-74). Totowa, NJ: Allanheld, Osmun.

Elian, M. and Dean, G. (1983). Need for and use of social and health service by multiple sclerosis patients living at the home in England. *Lancet, 1* (whole no. 8333), 1091-1093.

Evans, R., Fox, H., Pritzl, D., and Halar, E. (1984). Group treatment of physically disabled adults by telephone. *Social Work in Health Care, 9*(3), 77-84.

Foster, Z. and Mendel, S. (1979). Mutual help groups for patients: Taking steps toward change. *Health and Social Work, 4*(3), 82-98.

Frey, D., Oman, K., Robins, J., and Smith, E. J. (1991). Psychiatric home health care for AIDS patients. *Journal of Home Health Care Practice, 3*(3), 34-45.

Friedman, D., Hawkins, D. W., and Wright, A. R. (1994). 20 hot job tracks. *U.S. News & World Report, 117*(17), 110-122.

Gelman, S. (1986). Life vs. death: The value of ethical uncertainty. *Health and Social Work, 11*(2), 118-125.

Gill, G. M. (1991). Social work intervention with stroke patients and their families. *Journal of Home Health Care Practice, 4*(1), 57-62.

Glaser, B. G. and Strauss, A. L. (1967). *The discovery of grounded theory.* Chicago: Aldine.

Goldstein, M. K. (1989). Physicians and teams. In R. Hemm (Ed.), *Geriatric medicine annual.* Oradell, NJ: Medical Economic Books.

Goode, R. (1992). *Medical social work standards for home health care practice.* Unpublished workshop notes. Columbus, Ohio.

Griff, S. L. and Lerman, D. (1987). The future of home care. In D. Lerman (Ed.), *Home care: Positioning the hospital for the future* (pp. 265-271). Chicago: American Hospital Publishing, Inc.

Health Care Financing Administration. (1990, June). *Medicare home health agency manual* (Publication No. 11, §234.9). Washington, DC: U.S. Government Printing Office.

Health Care Financing Administration. (1992). *The HCFA Review, 13*(4), p. 40.

Kane, R. (1985). Health policy and social workers in health: Present and future. *Health and Social Work, 10*(4), 258-270.

Kaye, L. (1992). *Home health care.* Newbury Park, CA: Sage.

Kempen, G. I. and Suurmeijer, T. P. (1991). Factors influencing professional home care utilization among the elderly. *Social Sciences Medicine, 32*(1), 77-81.

Krausz, S. (1980). Group psychotherapy with legally blind patients. *Clinical Social Work Journal, 1*(8), 37-49.

Kruse, E. A. and Wood, M. (1989). Delivering mental health services in the home: Community home health care. *Caring, 8*(6), 28-29, 32-34, 59.

Lee, S. (1980). Interdisciplinary teaming in primary care: A process of evolution and resolution. *Social Work in Health Care, 5*(3), 237-244.

Lerman, D. (Ed.) (1987). *Home care: Positioning the hospital for the future.* Chicago: American Hospital Publishing, Inc.

Levande, D. I., Bowden, S. W., and Mollema, J. (1987). Home health services for dependent elders: The social work dimension. *Journal of Gerontological Social Work, 11*(3/4), 5-17.

Lindenberg, R. E. and Coulton, C. (1980). Planning for post-hospital care: A follow-up study. *Health and Social Work, 5*(1), 45-50.

Lindner, A. L. (1987). Bringing the hospital home. *University Hospital, 5*(1) (Cleveland, OH).

Lowe, J. I. and Herranen, M. (1978). Conflict in teamwork: Understanding roles and relationships. *Social Work in Health Care, 3*(3), 232-240.

Lurie, A., Pinskey, S., and Tuzman, L. (1981). Training social workers in discharge planning. *Health and Social Work, 6*(4), 12-18.

McAllister, J. C. III, Black, B. L., Griffin, R. E., and Smith, J. E. (1986). Controversial issues in home health care: A roundtable discussion. *American Journal of Hospital Pharmacy, 43*(4), 933-946.

McCann, B. A. and The Joint Commission on Accreditation of Hospitals Home Care Project (1987, September 14). *Assessing home care quality (Issue brief no. 474)*. Washington, DC: The George Washington University.

Naisbitt, J. L. (1988). *Megatrends*. New York: Warner Books.

NASW (1991). *Social work speaks*, Second edition. Silver Spring, MD: National Association of Social Workers.

National Association of Home Care (1999). *Home health care stats*. For consumers. Washington, DC: Author. <www.NAHC.org>.

Noble, J. Jr. and Conley, R. (1982). Cost containment. In D. Lum (Ed.), *Social work and health care policy* (pp. 151-176). Totowa, NJ: Allanheld, Osmun.

Ohio Council for Home Care (1997). *The 1997 resource guide*. Columbus, OH: Author.

Ohio Department of Health. (1992). *The 1991 home health care registration report*. Columbus, OH: Author.

Olson, H. and Mintun, G. (1990, January). Capturing new human services markets. *Caring, 9*(1), pp. 16-17, 42-43.

Parker, M. (1990, January). How to succeed in the home care business in the 1990s. *Caring 9*(1), pp. 8-10, 12-14.

Parry, J. (1980). Group services for the chronically ill and disabled. *Social Work with Groups, 3*(1), 59-61.

Pendarvis, J. and Grinnell, R. (1980). The use of a rehabilitation team for stroke patients. *Social Work in Health Care, 6*(2), 77-86.

Pesznecker, B. L. and Paquin, R. (1982). Implementing interdisciplinary team practice in home care of geriatric clients. *Journal of Gerontological Nursing, 8*(9), 504-508.

Poole, D. and Carlton, T. (1986). A model for analyzing utilization of maternal and child health services. *Health and Social Work, 11*(3), 209-222.

Reamer, F. (1985). The emergency of bioethics in social work. *Health Care and Social Work, 10*(4), 271-281.

Roy, C., Flynn, E., and Atcherson, E. (1982). Group sessions for home homodialysis assistants. *Health and Social Work, 71*(1), 65-71.

Roy, P. and Sumpter, H. (1983). Group social work for the recently bereaved. *Health and Social Work, 8*(3), 230.

Sandman, G. (1981). Discharge planning: A social worker's perspective. In K. M. McKeehan (Ed.), *Continuing care: A multi-disciplinary approach to discharge* (pp. 107-118). St. Louis, MO: C. V. Mosby.

Schrager, J., Halman, M., Myens, D., Nichols, R., and Rosenberg, L. (1978). Impediment to the course and effectiveness of discharge planning. *Social Work in Health Care, 4*(1), 65-79.

Schreiber, H. (1981). Discharge planning: Key to the future of hospital social work. *Health and Social Work, 6*(2), 48-53.

Shibbal-Champagne, S. and Lipinska-Stachow, D. (1985-1986). Alzheimer's educational/support group: Considerations for success-awareness of family tasks, pre-planning, and active professional facilitation. *Journal of Gerontological Social Work, 9*(2), 41-48.

Soldo, B. and Manton, G. (1985). Health status and service needs of the older old: Current patterns and future trends. *Milbank Memorial Fund, 63*(2), 286-319.

Spring, J. (1981). Medicare: An advocacy perspective. *Social Work in Health Care, 6*(4), 77-89.

Tamme, P. (1985). Abuse of the adult client in home care. *Family and Community Health, 8*(2), 54-65.

Thoebaben, M. (1988). Nurse/social worker home care. *Home Healthcare Nurse, 6*(1), 37-39.

Thoebaben, M. and Woodward, W. (1991). The psychosomatic needs of home-bound cardiac patients and families. *Journal of Home Health Care Practice, 4*(1), 22-30.

Wattenberg, S. and McGann, L. (1984). Medicare or medigap: Dilemmas for the elderly. *Health and Social Work, 9*(3), 229-237.

Watts, R. (1967, April). Medicare and the hospital based social worker. *Hospitals, 41*, 74-81.

Wilcox, J. A. and Tabu, M. A. (1991). Informal helpers of elderly home care clients. *Health and Social Work, 16*(4), 258-265.

Williams, S. D. and Williams, J. R. (1988). *How to market home health care services.* Albany, NY: Delmar.

Wilson, S. A. (1989). The ethnography of death, dying, and hospice care. Unpublished doctoral dissertation, The University of Wisconsin, Milwaukee.

Zink, M. R. (1987). A tool for holistic care assessment of the older patient. *The Older Patient, 1*(9), 29-31.

Zink, M. R. and Bissonnette, A. (1990). A unique multi-disciplinary approach to urban geriatric home care. *Nursing Administration Quarterly, 14*(2), 69-73.

Index

Printed in the United States
by Baker & Taylor Publisher Services